SKILLMASTERS

3-Minute
Assessment

SECOND EDITION

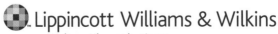

Lippincott Williams & Wilkins
a Wolters Kluwer business
Philadelphia · Baltimore · New York · London
Buenos Aires · Hong Kong · Sydney · Tokyo

Staff

Executive Publisher
Judith A. Schilling McCann, RN, MSN

Editorial Director
William J. Kelly

Clinical Director
Joan M. Robinson, RN, MSN

Senior Art Director
Arlene Putterman

Clinical Manager
Collette Bishop Hendler, RN, BS, CCRN

Editorial Project Manager
Sean Webb

Clinical Project Manager
Cynthia L. Brophy, RN, BSN, CPAN

Editor
Patricia Nale

Copy Editors
Kimberly Bilotta (supervisor), Jen Fielding,
Laura Healy, Pamela Wingrod

Designers
Jan Greenberg (project manager)

Digital Composition Services
Diane Paluba (manager),
Joyce Rossi Biletz, Donna S. Morris

Manufacturing
Beth J. Welsh

Editorial Assistants
Megan L. Aldinger, Karen J. Kirk,
Linda K. Ruhf

Design Assistant
Georg W. Purvis IV

Indexer
Deborah Tourtlotte

S3MA021209

FOCUS CHARTING is a registered trademark of
Creative Healthcare Management Inc.

**Library of Congress
Cataloging-in-Publication Data**

Skillmasters. 3-minute assessment. —2nd ed.
　　p. ; cm.
　Includes bibliographical references and index.
　1. Nursing assessment—Handbooks, manuals, etc.
　I. Lippincott Williams & Wilkins. II. Title: 3-minute
assessment. III. Title: Three-minute assessment.
[DNLM: 1. Nursing Assessment—methods.
　2. Medical History Taking—methods.
　WY 100.4 S628 2006]
　　RT48 .S58 2006
　616.07'5—dc22
ISBN 1-58255-864-7 (alk. paper)　　　　2006014462

Contents

Contributors and consultants

Katrina D. Allen, RN, MSN, CCRN
ADN Nursing Instructor
Faulkner State Community College
Bay Minette, Ala.

Beverly Anderson, RN, MSN
Associate Professor
Malcolm X College
Chicago

Kim Cooper, RN, MSN
Nursing Department Program Chair
Ivy Tech Community College of Indiana
Terre Haute

Ellie Z. Franges, RN, MSN, CRNP, CNRN
Nurse Practitioner, Neurosurgery
St. Luke's Hospital & Health Network
Bethlehem, Pa.

Rhonda J. Gall, MSN, APRN, BC, GNP
Faculty/Lecturer
Bowie (Md.) State University

Ann S. McQueen, RNC, MSN, CRNP
Family Nurse Practitioner
Health Link Medical Center
Southampton, Pa.

Catherine Pence, RN, MSN, CCRN
Assistant Professor
Northern Kentucky University
Highland Heights

Catherine Shields, RN, BSN
Nursing Instructor
Ocean County Vocational-Technical School
 of Nursing
Lakehurst, N.J.

Beth Spence, RN, CEN, CFRN, EMT-P
Critical Care Transport Nurse/Flight Nurse,
 ER Nurse
Sunstar
Largo, Fla.

Allison J. Terry, RN, PhD
Director of Community Certification,
 Mental Retardation Division
State of Alabama Department of Mental
 Health
Montgomery

Karen Zulkowski, RN, DNS, CWS
Associate Professor
Montana State University
Billings

Guide to *SkillMasters*: 3-Minute Assessment

SkillMasters: 3-Minute Assessment, Second Edition, concisely explains how to assess patients with a particular complaint within 3 minutes and how to perform an accurate, rapid assessment of each body system. This manual can be useful to both practicing nurses and student nurses in any setting.

Chapter 1 of *SkillMasters: 3-Minute Assessment* is on obtaining a health history. It includes tips for better interviewing and essential questions to ask about each body system. Basic physical assessment techniques and information on performing a general survey of the patient are also covered. Chapter 2 highlights rapid assessment components, including an across-the-life-span perspective. Chapter 3 is a new chapter on documentation that includes information on documentation systems, rules of charting, and legal implications.

Chapters 4 through 14 focus on the individual body systems, starting with the respiratory system. Each chapter includes a brief description of the body system's anatomy and physiology, followed by a guide for performing a physical assessment of the system using inspection, palpation, percussion, and auscultation. For each physical assessment component, there's a discussion of normal and abnormal findings.

KEY FEATURES

As a new feature in this edition, the *Guidelines for a 3-minute assessment* section in each chapter has been highlighted for easy access. Also new to this edition is an appendix on domestic abuse assessment.

Each body system chapter focuses on common chief complaints and helps you explore them with a relevant history and physical examination. Each of these chapters also shows you how to analyze the data. Pediatric and geriatric tips are emphasized in age-related situations.

Throughout the text, prominent symbols highlight recurring information. *A closer look* shows typical anatomic structures, and *Checklist* describes normal assessment findings. On charts for each body system, *Diagnostic impression* presents associated signs and symptoms under their possible causes to help you focus your assessment.

Each chapter ends with *SkillCheck,* a self-quiz for you to test your knowledge of the information presented and your ability to apply that knowledge in various scenarios. The quizzes help you identify your strengths and enable you to concentrate on those areas where you need improvement.

Basic assessment review

Obtaining a health history and performing a physical assessment are essential steps of nursing assessment. Knowing how to complete these steps will help you uncover significant problems and establish an appropriate care plan. Although doing a complete health history and physical assessment can be time-consuming, doing them in a systematic fashion will help you perform a 3-minute assessment when your patient develops symptoms. This chapter presents the basics of taking a health history and performing a physical assessment, which lay the groundwork for performing a 3-minute assessment of symptoms.

Any assessment involves collecting two kinds of data: objective and subjective. Objective data are obtained through hearing, touching, smelling and seeing, and are verifiable—for example, a red swollen arm in a patient who is experiencing arm pain is data that can be seen and verified by someone other than the patient. Subjective data can't be verified by anyone other than the patient; they're gathered solely from the patient's own account—for example, "My head hurts" or "I have trouble sleeping at night."

Obtaining the health history

A health history is used to gather subjective data about the patient and to explore previous and current problems. First, ask the patient about his general physical and emotional health, and then ask him questions about specific body systems and structures.

The accuracy and completeness of your patient's answers largely depend on your skill as an interviewer. Before you start asking questions, review the communication guidelines in the following sections.

INTERVIEWING THE PATIENT

Before asking your first question, you need to set the stage—specifically, explain to the patient what you'll cover during the interview and establish rapport with him. Here's how:
- Choose a quiet, private, well-lit interview setting away from distractions. Such a setting will make it easier for you and your patient to interact and will help the patient feel more at ease.
- Make sure the patient is comfortable. Sit facing him, 3′ to 4′ (1 to 1.5 m) away.
- Introduce yourself and explain that the purpose of the health history and assessment is to identify his problem

and provide information for planning care.

■ Reassure the patient that everything he says will be kept confidential.

■ Tell the patient how long the interview will last and ask him what he expects from it.

■ Use touch sparingly. Many people aren't comfortable with strangers hugging, patting, or touching them.

■ Assess the patient to see if language barriers exist. For instance, does he speak and understand English?

■ Assess the patient to see if communication barriers exist. Can he see you or hear you? Find out his preferred method of communicating.

■ Most facilities have a bank of interpreters available to assist with English translations or sign language, or a member of the patient's family may be helpful for interpretation.

■ If your patient is hearing impaired, make sure the area is well lit, face him, and speak slowly and clearly so that he can read your lips.

■ During your assessment, speak slowly and clearly, using easy-to-understand language. Avoid medical terms and jargon.

■ Address the patient by a formal name, such as Mr. Jones or Ms. Carter. Don't call him by his first name unless he asks you to. Treating the patient with respect encourages him to trust you and provide accurate and complete information.

■ Listen attentively and make eye contact frequently. However, be aware that patients from different cultures—including Native Americans, Asians, and those from Arabic-speaking countries—may find eye contact disrespectful or aggressive.

■ Use reassuring gestures, such as nodding your head, to encourage the patient to keep talking.

■ Watch for nonverbal cues that indicate the patient is uncomfortable or unsure about how to answer a question. For example, he might lower his voice or glance around uneasily.

■ Be aware of your own nonverbal cues that might cause the patient to "clam up" or become defensive. For example, if you cross your arms, you might appear "closed off" from him. If you stand while he's sitting, you might appear superior. If you glance at your watch, you might appear bored or rushed, which could keep him from answering questions completely.

Observe the patient closely to see if he understands each question. If he doesn't appear to understand, repeat the question using different words or familiar examples. For instance, instead of asking, "Did you have respiratory difficulty after exercising?" ask "Did you have to sit down after walking around the block?"

You might also use a different type of question. An open-ended question such as "How did you fall?" lets the patient respond more freely. The response can provide answers to many other questions.

For instance, from the patient's answer, you might learn that he has fallen before, that he was unsteady on his feet, and that he fell before dinner. Armed with this information, you might deduce that he had a syncopal episode caused by hypoglycemia.

You can also ask closed questions, which are unlikely to provide extra information but might encourage the patient to give clear, concise feedback. (See *Two ways to ask questions*.)

Communication strategies

In addition to the tips listed previously, the following communication techniques—silence, facilitation, confirmation, reflection, clarification, summary, and conclusion—can help you make the most of your patient interview.

SILENCE

Moments of silence during the interview encourage the patient to continue talking and give you a chance to assess his ability to organize thoughts. You may find this technique difficult (most people are uncomfortable with silence), but the more you use it, the more comfortable you'll become.

FACILITATION

Facilitation encourages the patient to continue with his story. Using such phrases as "please continue," "go on," or even, "uh-huh," show him that you're interested in what he's saying.

CONFIRMATION

Confirmation ensures that you and the patient are on the same track. You might say, "If I understand you correctly, you said…" and then repeat the information the patient gave. This technique helps clear up misconceptions you or the patient might have.

REFLECTION

Reflection—or repeating something the patient has just said—can help you obtain more specific information. For example, a patient with a stomachache might say, "I know I have an ulcer." You might repeat, "You know you have an ulcer?" And the patient might then say, "Yes. I had one before and the pain is the same."

Two ways to ask questions

Questions can be characterized as either open-ended or closed.

Open-ended questions
Open-ended questions require the patient to express feelings, opinions, and ideas. They also help you gather more information than can be gathered with closed questions. Open-ended questions encourage a good nurse-patient rapport because they show that you're interested in what the patient has to say. Examples of such questions include:
• What prompted you to seek care tonight?
• How would you describe the problems you're having with your breathing?
• What lung problems, if any, do other members of your family have?

Closed questions
Closed questions can be answered with a "yes" or "no" or a one- or two-word response. They limit the development of nurse-patient rapport. Closed questions can help you "zoom in" on specific points, but they don't provide the patient the opportunity to elaborate. Examples of closed questions include:
• Do you ever get short of breath?
• Are you the only one in your family with lung problems?

CLARIFICATION

Clarification is used to clear up confusing, vague, or misunderstood information. For example, if your patient says, "I can't stand this," your response might be, "What can't you stand?" or

"What do you mean by 'I can't stand this?'" This gives the patient an opportunity to explain the statement.

SUMMARY

Summarizing, or restating, the information the patient gave you ensures that the data you've collected is accurate and complete. Summarizing also signals that the interview is about to end.

CONCLUSION

Signaling the patient that you're ready to conclude the interview provides him the opportunity to gather his thoughts and make final pertinent statements. You can do this verbally by saying, "I think I have all the information I need now. Is there anything you'd like to add?"

Specific questions to ask

Asking the right questions is a critical part of any interview. To obtain a complete health history, gather information from each of the following categories, in sequence:

1. biographic data
2. chief complaint
3. medical history
4. allergy history
5. family history
6. psychosocial history
7. activities of daily living.

BIOGRAPHIC DATA

Start the health history by obtaining biographic information from the patient. Do this first so you don't forget about this information after you become involved in details of the patient's health. Ask the patient for his name, address, telephone number, birth date, age, marital status, religion, and nationality. Find out who he lives with and the

name and telephone number of a person to contact in case of an emergency.

Also, ask the patient about his health care, including who his primary practitioner is and how he gets to the practitioner's office. Ask if he has ever been treated before for his present problem.

Your patient's answers to basic questions can offer important clues about personality, medical problems, and reliability. If he can't provide accurate information, ask him for the name of a friend or relative who can. Document who gave you the information.

CHIEF COMPLAINT

Try to pinpoint why the patient is seeking care at this time. Document this information in the patient's exact words to avoid misinterpretation. Ask him what his symptoms are and when they developed, what prompted him to seek medical attention, and how the symptoms have affected his life and ability to function. His chief complaint will be the basis for your 3-minute assessment.

MEDICAL HISTORY

Ask the patient about past and current medical problems, such as hypertension, diabetes, or back pain. Typical questions include:

■ Have you ever been hospitalized? If so, when and for what reason?

■ Which childhood illnesses did you have?

■ Are you undergoing treatment for anything? If so, what's the treatment for and who's your physician?

■ Have you ever had surgery? If so, when and for what reason?

■ Do you have pain? Have you had pain in the past or do you have ongoing pain? If so, tell me about the pain. Where is it? On a scale of 0 to 10 with 10 being the worst, how bad is the pain? How long have you had the pain? What relieves it or makes it worse? Are you taking medications for it?

■ Are you taking medications, including over-the-counter preparations, such as aspirin, vitamins, or cough syrup? If so, how much do you take and how often? Do you use home remedies such as homemade ointments? Do you use herbal preparations or take dietary supplements? Do you use other alternative therapies, such as acupuncture, therapeutic massage, or chiropractic therapy?

ALLERGY HISTORY

Ask about allergies or reactions the patient has had. Note the type and severity of reactions. Common allergies include environmental and seasonal allergies as well as sensitivities to tape, latex, food—for example, shellfish, medications, and blood. Typical questions include:

■ Have you ever had an allergic reaction to anything, such as a food, rubber gloves, or medication you have taken?

■ What was your reaction?

■ Did you develop an upset stomach, rash, or difficulty breathing?

■ Did the reaction require medical treatment?

Document the allergy and the reaction the patient experienced, and follow your facility's policy and procedure for documenting allergies in the patient's chart.

FAMILY HISTORY

Questioning the patient about his family's health is a good way to uncover whether he's at risk for certain illnesses. Typical questions include:

■ Are your mother, father, and siblings living? If not, how old were they when

they died? What was the cause of death?

■ If they're alive, do they have asthma, cancer, cataracts, diabetes, glaucoma, heart disease, hemophilia, high blood pressure, sickle cell anemia, stroke, renal disease, tuberculosis, or other illnesses?

PSYCHOSOCIAL HISTORY

Find out how the patient feels about himself, his place in society, and his relationships with others. Ask about occupation, education, financial status, responsibilities, and abuse. This information will help you understand the patient's personality, coping mechanisms, lifestyle, and financial status. Typical questions include:

■ How have you coped with medical or emotional crises in the past?

■ Have you had significant life changes recently? Have you noticed changes in your personality or behavior?

■ Is the emotional support you receive from family and friends adequate?

■ How close do you live to health care facilities and are they easy to get to?

■ Do you have health insurance?

■ Are you on a fixed income with no extra money for health care?

■ Do you ever feel threatened at home? (See *Asking about abuse,* page 6.)

ACTIVITIES OF DAILY LIVING

Find out what's normal for the patient by asking him to describe a typical day. Include the following areas in your assessment: diet and elimination; exercise and sleep; work and leisure; use of tobacco, alcohol, and other drugs; and religious observances.

Diet and elimination. Ask the patient about his appetite, special diets,

Asking about abuse

Anyone can be a victim of abuse: a boyfriend or girlfriend, a spouse, an elderly patient, a child, or a parent. Also, abuse can come in many forms: physical, psychological, emotional, and sexual. When taking a health history, ask two open-ended questions: When do you feel safe at home? When don't you feel safe?

Watching the reaction
Even when you don't immediately suspect an abusive situation, be aware of how your patient reacts to open-ended questions. Is the patient defensive, hostile, confused, or frightened? Assess how he interacts with you and others. Does he seem withdrawn or frightened or show other inappropriate behavior? Keep his reactions in mind when you perform your physical assessment.

and food allergies. Can he afford to buy enough food? Who at his house cooks and shops? Also ask about frequency of bowel movements and laxative use. When was his last bowel movement and was it normal?

Exercise and sleep. Ask the patient if he follows an exercise program; if so, have him describe it. Ask how many hours he sleeps at night, what his sleep pattern is like, and whether he feels rested after sleep.

Work and leisure. Ask the patient what he does for a living and what he does during leisure time. Does he have hobbies?

Use of tobacco, alcohol, and other drugs. Ask the patient if he smokes cigarettes or chews tobacco. If so, how much does he smoke or chew each

day? Does he drink alcohol? If so, how many drinks each day? Ask if he uses illicit drugs, such as marijuana or cocaine. If so, how often?

A patient may understate the amount he drinks because of embarrassment. If you're having trouble getting him to give you an honest estimate, try overestimating the amount. For example, you might say, "You told me you drink beer. Do you drink about a six-pack a day?" The patient's response might be, "No, I drink about half that."

Religious observances. Ask the patient if he has religious beliefs that affect diet, dress, or health practices. Patients will feel reassured when you make it clear that you understand these points.

Professional outlook
Be nonjudgmental and maintain a professional, neutral approach, and don't offer advice. For example, don't suggest that the patient enter a drug rehabilitation program. That type of response will put him on the defensive and may make him reluctant to answer subsequent questions honestly.

Also, avoid unwanted advice. Statements such as, "The physician knows what's best for you" make the patient feel inferior and break down communication. Finally, don't use leading or biased questions such as "You don't do drugs, do you?" to get the answer you're hoping for. This type of question, based on your own values, will make the patient feel guilty and might prevent him from responding honestly.

REVIEWING STRUCTURES AND SYSTEMS
The last part of the health history is a systematic assessment of the patient's

body structures and systems. Always start at the top of the head and work your way down the body. This helps ensure that you cover every area. When questioning an elderly patient, remember that he may have difficulty hearing or communicating. (See *Overcoming communication problems with elderly patients.*)

Asking the right questions

Information gained from a health history forms the basis for your care plan, enabling you to distinguish physical changes and devise a holistic approach to treatment. As with other nursing skills, your interviewing technique will improve only with practice, practice, and more practice.

Here are some key questions to ask your patient about each body structure and system.

HEAD

Do you get headaches or dizzy? If so, where's the pain located and how intense is it? How often do the headaches occur, and how long do they last? Does anything trigger them, and how do you relieve them? Describe your dizziness. Have you ever passed out? Have you ever had a head injury? Do you have lumps or bumps on your head?

EYES, EARS, NOSE

When was your last eye examination? Do you wear glasses? Do you have glaucoma, cataracts, or color blindness? Does light bother your eyes? Do you have excessive tearing; blurred vision; double vision; or dry, itchy, burning, inflamed, or swollen eyes?

Do you have loss of balance, ringing in your ears, deafness, or poor hearing? Have you ever had ear surgery? If so,

> ## Overcoming communication problems with elderly patients
>
> An elderly patient may have sensory impairment, impaired memory, or a decreased attention span. If your patient is confused or has trouble communicating, you may need to rely on a family member for some or all of the health history.

why and when? Do you wear a hearing aid? Do you have pain, swelling, or discharge from your ears? If so, has this problem occurred before and how frequently?

Have you ever had nasal surgery? If so, why and when? Do you have difficulty with smell? Have you ever had sinusitis or nosebleeds? Do you have nasal problems that cause breathing difficulties, frequent sneezing, or discharge?

MOUTH AND THROAT

Do you have mouth sores, a dry mouth, loss of taste, a toothache, or bleeding gums? Do you wear dentures, and do they fit?

Do you have a sore throat, fever, or chills? How often do you get a sore throat, and have you seen a physician for this?

Do you have difficulty swallowing? If so, is the problem with solids or liquids? Is it a constant problem or does it accompany sore throat or another problem? What, if anything, makes it go away?

NECK

Do you have swelling, soreness, lack of movement, stiffness, or pain in your neck? If so, did something specific cause it to happen such as too much exercise? How long have you had the problem? Does anything relieve it or aggravate it?

RESPIRATORY SYSTEM

Do you have shortness of breath on exertion or while lying in bed? How many pillows do you use at night? Do you have pain or wheezing when breathing? Do you have a productive cough? If so, describe the sputum. How much is it? What color is it? Is it blood tinged? Do you have night sweats?

Have you ever been treated for pneumonia, asthma, emphysema, or frequent respiratory tract infections? Have you ever had a chest X-ray or a tuberculin skin test? If so, when, and what were the results?

CARDIOVASCULAR SYSTEM

Do you have chest pain, palpitations, irregular heartbeat, fast heartbeat, shortness of breath, or a persistent cough? If so, under what circumstances? Have you ever had an electrocardiogram? If so, when?

Do you have high blood pressure, peripheral vascular disease, swelling of the ankles and hands, varicose veins, cold extremities, or intermittent pain in your legs?

BREASTS

Ask women these questions: Do you perform monthly breast self-examinations? Have you noticed a lump, a change in breast contour, breast pain, or discharge from your nipples? Have you ever had breast cancer? Has any-

one else in your family had it? Have you ever had a mammogram? When, and what were the results?

Ask men these questions: Do you have pain in your breast tissue? Have you noticed lumps or a change in contour?

GASTROINTESTINAL SYSTEM

Have you had nausea, vomiting, loss of appetite, heartburn, abdominal pain, frequent belching, or passing of gas? Have you lost or gained weight recently? How frequent are your bowel movements, and what color, odor, and consistency are your stools? Have you noticed a change in your regular pattern? Do you use antacids or laxatives frequently?

Have you had hemorrhoids, rectal bleeding, hernias, gallbladder disease, or a liver disease such as hepatitis?

URINARY SYSTEM

Do you have urinary problems, such as burning during urination, incontinence, frequency, urgency, retention, reduced urinary flow, straining, or dribbling? Do you get up during the night to urinate? If so, how many times? What color is your urine, and do you notice an odor? Have you ever noticed blood in it? Have you been treated for kidney stones or kidney disease?

REPRODUCTIVE SYSTEM

Ask women these questions: How old were you when you started menstruating? How often do you get your period, and how long does it usually last? Do you have clots or pain? If you're perimenopausal, what symptoms are you experiencing? If you're postmenopausal, at what age did you stop menstruating and do you experience postmenopausal bleeding? Have you ever been pregnant? If so, how many times? What was the method of delivery? How many pregnancies resulted in live births? How many were miscarriages? Have you ever had an abortion?

Do you practice or use birth control? What's your method of birth control? Are you in a long-term, monogamous relationship? Have you ever had a vaginal infection or a sexually transmitted disease? Do you have vaginal discharge or odor? When was your last gynecologic examination and Papanicolaou test? What were the results?

Ask men these questions: Have you ever had a prostate examination and, if so, when? Do you perform monthly testicular self-examinations? Have you noticed penile pain, discharge, or lesions or testicular lumps? Do you use birth control? Have you had a vasectomy? Are you in a long-term, monogamous relationship? Have you ever had a sexually transmitted disease?

You may need to investigate sexual orientation if appropriate and warranted. If the patient is not in a long-term monogamous relationship, ask if he practices safe, protected sex. Has he ever been tested for HIV infection? What were the results? Would he like to be tested? Ensure confidentiality.

MUSCULOSKELETAL SYSTEM

Do you have difficulty or pain when walking, sitting, or standing? Are you steady on your feet, or do you lose your balance easily? Do you have arthritis, gout, a back injury, muscle weakness, or paralysis?

NEUROLOGIC SYSTEM

Have you ever had dizziness, blackouts, or seizures? Do you ever experience tremors, twitching, numbness, tingling, or loss of sensation in a part of your body? Have you noticed changes or experienced memory loss?

ENDOCRINE SYSTEM

Have you been unusually tired lately? Do you feel hungry or thirsty more than usual? Have you lost weight for unexplained reasons? How well can you tolerate heat or cold? Have you noticed changes in your hair texture or color? Have you been losing hair? Do you take hormonal medications?

HEMATOLOGIC SYSTEM

Have you ever been diagnosed with anemia or another blood abnormality? Do you bruise easily or have prolonged bleeding with cuts? Have you ever had a blood transfusion? If so, have you ever had a reaction to the blood?

EMOTIONAL STATUS

Do you ever experience mood swings or memory loss? Do you ever feel anxious, depressed, or unable to concentrate? Are you feeling unusually stressed? Do you ever feel unable to cope?

Performing the physical assessment

After you've taken the patient's health history, proceed to the hands-on part of the assessment. During the physical assessment, you'll use all of your senses and a systematic approach to collect information about your patient's health.

As you proceed through the physical assessment, you can also teach your patient about his body, which will help

Assessment tools

Tools used for assessment include:
- blood pressure cuff
- cotton balls
- gloves
- metric ruler (clear)
- near-vision and visual acuity charts
- ophthalmoscope
- otoscope
- penlight
- percussion hammer
- safety pins
- scale with height measurement
- skin calipers
- specula (nasal and vaginal)
- stethoscope
- tape measure (cloth or paper)
- thermometer
- tuning fork
- wooden tongue blade.

develop rapport. For instance, you can explain how to do a testicular self-examination or why the patient should monitor a mole.

More than anything else, successful assessment requires critical thinking. How does one finding fit in with the big picture? An initial assessment guides your whole care plan.

COLLECTING THE TOOLS

Before starting a physical assessment, assemble the necessary tools. (See *Assessment tools*.)

Use a stethoscope with a diaphragm and a bell. The diaphragm has a flat, thin, plastic surface that picks up high-pitched sounds such as breath sounds. The bell has a smaller, open end that picks up low-pitched sounds, such as third and fourth heart sounds.

You'll need a penlight to illuminate the inside of the patient's nose and mouth, cast tangential light on lesions, and evaluate pupillary reactions. An ophthalmoscope enables you to examine the internal structures of the eye; an otoscope, the external auditory canal and tympanic membrane.

Other tools include cotton balls and safety pins to test sensation and pain differentiation, a percussion hammer to evaluate deep tendon reflexes, and gloves to protect the patient and you from potential body fluid exposure. Consider latex allergy when choosing gloves.

PERFORMING A GENERAL SURVEY

After assembling the necessary tools, move on to the first part of the physical assessment: forming initial impressions of the patient, preparing him for the assessment, and obtaining baseline data, including height, weight, and vital signs. This information will direct the rest of your assessment.

Forming initial impressions

A patient's behavior, mobility, and physical appearance can offer subtle clues about his health. Carefully observe him for unusual behavior or signs of illness.

Preparing the patient

If possible, introduce yourself to the patient before the assessment, preferably when he's dressed. Meeting him under less-threatening circumstances will decrease his anxiety when you perform the assessment.

Keep in mind that the patient may be worried that you'll find a problem. He may also consider the assessment an invasion of privacy because you're observing and touching sensitive, private and, perhaps, painful body areas.

Before you start, briefly explain what you're planning to do, why you're doing it, how long it will take, what position changes it will require, and what equipment you'll use. As you perform the assessment, explain each step in detail. A well-prepared patient won't be surprised or feel unexpected discomfort, so he'll trust you more and cooperate better.

Put your patient at ease, but know where to draw the line. Maintain professionalism during the examination. Humor can help put the patient at ease, but avoid sarcasm and keep jokes in good taste.

When you're finished with your assessment, allow the patient to get dressed. Document your findings in a short, concise paragraph. Include only essential information that communicates your overall impression of the patient. For example, if your patient has a lesion, simply note that fact. You'll describe the lesion in detail when you complete the physical assessment.

Obtaining baseline data

Accurate measurements of your patient's height, weight, and vital signs provide critical information about the patient's body functions.

The first time you assess a patient, record baseline vital signs and statistics. Afterward, take measurements at regular intervals, depending on the patient's condition and your facility's policy. A series of readings usually provides more valuable information than a single set. If you obtain an abnormal value, take the vital sign again to make sure it's accurate. Remember that nor-

mal readings vary with the patient's age and from patient to patient (an abnormal value for one patient may be a normal value for another).

HEIGHT AND WEIGHT

Height and weight are important for evaluating nutritional status, calculating medication dosages, and assessing fluid loss or gain. Take the patient's baseline height and weight so you can gauge future weight changes or calculate medication dosages in an emergency. Keep this information handy so you can refer to it quickly, if needed. (See *Measuring height and weight*, page 12.)

BODY TEMPERATURE

Body temperature is measured in degrees Fahrenheit (F) or degrees Celsius (C). Normal body temperature ranges from 96.7° to 100.5° F (35.9° to 38° C), depending on the route used for measurement.

Hyperthermia describes an oral temperature above 104° F (40° C); hypothermia describes a rectal temperature below 95° F (35° C).

The conversion formula for Fahrenheit and Celsius are:

$$°C = (°F - 32) \div 1.8$$
$$°F = (°C \times 1.8) + 32$$

(See *Comparing temperature readings*, page 13.)

PULSE

The patient's pulse reflects the blood ejected with each heartbeat. To assess the pulse, palpate one of the patient's arterial pulse points and note the rate, rhythm, and amplitude (strength) of the pulse. A normal pulse for an adult is between 60 and 100 beats/minute.

Measuring height and weight

Have the patient remove his shoes and dress in a hospital gown. Then use these techniques to measure his height and weight.

Balancing the scale
Slide both weight bars on the scale to zero. The balancing arrow should stop in the center of the open box. If the scale has wheels, lock them before the patient gets on.

Measuring height
Ask the patient to get on the scale and turn his back to it. Move the height bar up over his head, and lift up the horizontal arm. Then lower the bar until the horizontal arm touches the top of his head. Now read the height measurement from the height bar.

Measuring weight
Slide the lower weight into the groove representing the largest increment below the patient's estimated weight. For example, if you think the patient weighs 145 lb (65.8 kg), slide the weight into the groove for 100 lb (45.4 kg).

Slide the upper weight across until the arrow on the right stops in the middle of the open box. If the arrow hits the bottom, slide the weight to a lower number. If the arrow hits the top, slide the weight to a higher number.

The patient's weight is the sum of these numbers. For example, if the lower weight is on 150 lb (68 kg) and the upper weight is on 12 lb (5.4 kg), the patient weighs 162 lb (73.5 kg).

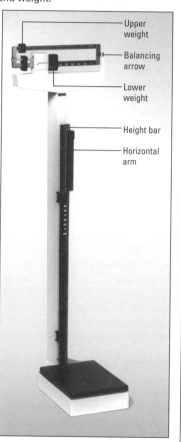

Labels: Upper weight; Balancing arrow; Lower weight; Height bar; Horizontal arm

---

The radial pulse is the most easily accessible pulse site. However, in cardiovascular emergencies, the femoral or carotid pulse may be more appropriate because these sites are larger and closer to the heart and more accurately reflect the heart's activity. (See *Locating pulse sites,* page 14.)

To palpate for a pulse, use the pads of your index and middle fingers. Press the area over the artery until you feel pulsations. If the rhythm is regular,

Comparing temperature readings

This chart compares the four different routes that can be used to take a patient's temperature.

Route	Normal temperature	Reading time	Used for
Oral	97.7° to 99.5° F (36.5° to 37.5° C)	3 to 5 minutes	Adults and older children who are awake, alert, oriented, and cooperative
Axillary (armpit)	96.7° to 98.5° F (35.9° to 36.9° C)	11 minutes	Patients with impaired immune systems in whom infection is a concern; less accurate because it can vary with blood flow to skin
Rectal	98.7° to 100.5° F (37° to 38° C)	2 minutes	Infants, young children, and confused or unconscious patients; wear gloves and lubricate the thermometer
Tympanic (ear)	98.2° to 100° F (36.8° to 37.8° C)	No set time; responds to subtle thermal changes and is unaffected by mouth breathing or patient movement	Adults and children, conscious and cooperative patients, and confused or unconscious patients; provides automatic timing through a push-button device

count the beats for 30 seconds and then multiply by 2 to get the number of beats per minute. If the rhythm is irregular or your patient has a pacemaker, auscultate the rate apically and count the beats for 60 seconds.

When taking the patient's pulse for the first time (or when obtaining baseline data), count the beats for 1 minute.

Avoid using your thumb to count the pulse because the thumb has a strong pulse of its own. If you need to palpate

the carotid arteries, avoid exerting a lot of pressure, which can stimulate the vagus nerve and cause reflex bradycardia. Also, don't palpate both carotid pulses at the same time. Putting pressure on both sides of the patient's neck can impair cerebral blood flow and function.

If your patient has an irregular pulse, do the following:
■ Evaluate whether the irregularity follows a pattern.

Locating pulse sites

You can assess your patient's pulse rate at several sites, including those shown in the illustration below.

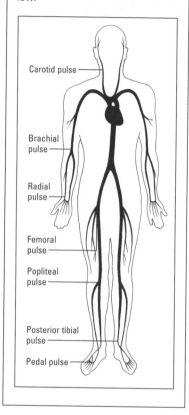

Carotid pulse

Brachial pulse

Radial pulse

Femoral pulse

Popliteal pulse

Posterior tibial pulse

Pedal pulse

diac contraction to eject sufficient blood into the peripheral circulation.

■ Assess pulse amplitude, or strength, using a numerical scale or descriptive term. Although numerical scales differ slightly between facilities, the following scale is commonly used:

Absent pulse: not palpable, measured as 0

Weak or thready pulse: hard to feel, easily obliterated by slight finger pressure, measured as +1

Normal pulse: easily palpable, obliterated by strong finger pressure, measured as +2

Increased pulse: measured as +3

Bounding pulse: readily palpable, forceful, not easily obliterated by pressure from the fingers, measured as +4.

RESPIRATIONS

Along with counting respirations, note the depth and rhythm of each breath. To determine the respiratory rate, count the number of respirations for 60 seconds. A rate of 10 to 20 breaths/minute is the normal range for an adult. If the patient knows you're counting how often he breathes, he may subconsciously alter the rate. To avoid this, count his respirations while you take his pulse.

Also, pay attention to the depth of the patient's respirations by watching his chest rise and fall; describe the breathing pattern. Is his breathing shallow, moderate, or deep? Observe the rhythm and symmetry of the chest wall as it expands during inspiration and relaxes during expiration. Be aware that skeletal deformity, broken ribs, and collapsed lung tissue can cause unequal chest expansion.

Use of accessory muscles can enhance lung expansion when oxygenation drops. Patients with chronic ob-

■ Auscultate the apical pulse while palpating the radial pulse. You should feel the pulse every time you hear a heartbeat.

■ Measure the pulse deficit — that is, the difference between the apical pulse rate and radial pulse rate. After you have this measurement, you can indirectly evaluate the ability of each car-

structive pulmonary disease (COPD) or respiratory distress may use accessory muscles, including the sternocleidomastoid muscles and abdominal muscles for breathing. Patient position during normal breathing may also suggest problems such as COPD. Normal respirations are quiet and easy, so note abnormal sounds, such as wheezing or stridor. Also note nasal flaring, pursed lip breathing, cyanosis, clubbing of fingers, or barrel chest.

BLOOD PRESSURE

Systolic and diastolic blood pressure readings are helpful in evaluating cardiac output, fluid and circulatory status, and arterial resistance. The systolic reading reflects the maximum pressure exerted on the arterial wall at the peak of left ventricular contraction. Normal systolic pressure ranges from 100 to 119 mm Hg.

The diastolic reading reflects the minimum pressure exerted on the arterial wall during left ventricular relaxation. This reading is generally more significant than the systolic reading because it evaluates arterial pressure when the heart is at rest. Normal diastolic pressure ranges from 60 to 79 mm Hg.

Patients with a systolic blood pressure of 120 to 139 mm Hg or diastolic blood pressure of 80 to 89 mm Hg are classified as "prehypertensive" and are at higher risk for hypertension. They should make lifestyle changes to prevent cardiovascular disease.

The sphygmomanometer, a device used to measure blood pressure, consists of an inflatable cuff, a pressure manometer, and a bulb with a valve. Correct cuff size is important to obtain an accurate reading. The bladder inside the cuff should encircle 80% of the arm's circumference in adults and 100% in children. To record a blood pressure, the cuff is centered over an artery, inflated, and deflated. (See *Using a sphygmomanometer,* page 16.)

As it deflates, listen with a stethoscope for Korotkoff's (clear tapping) sounds, which indicate the systolic and diastolic pressures. Blood pressure can be measured from most extremity pulse points. The brachial artery is used for most patients because of its accessibility. Avoid slow or repetitious blood pressure readings, allowing at least 15 seconds between readings.

If you have trouble hearing Korotkoff's sounds, try to intensify them by increasing vascular pressure below the cuff. Here are two techniques for doing this:
■ *Raising the arm.* Palpate the brachial pulse; mark its location with a pen to avoid losing the pulse spot. Apply the cuff and have the patient raise his arm above his head. Then inflate the cuff about 30 mm Hg above the patient's systolic pressure. Have him lower the arm until the cuff reaches heart level, deflate the cuff, and take a reading.
■ *Making a fist.* Position the patient's arm at heart level. Inflate the cuff to 30 mm Hg above the patient's systolic pressure, and ask him to make a fist. Have him rapidly open and close his hand 10 times; then deflate the cuff and take the reading.

PHYSICAL ASSESSMENT TECHNIQUES

During the physical assessment, use drapes, exposing only the area to be examined. Develop a pattern for your assessment, starting with the same body system and proceeding in the same sequence. Organize your steps to mini-

Using a sphygmomanometer

When using a sphygmomanometer, proper technique is essential for obtaining accurate and consistent results. Here are some helpful guidelines.

- Position your patient with his upper arm at heart level and his palm turned up.
- Apply the cuff snugly, 1″ (2.5 cm) above the brachial pulse, as shown in the top photo.
- Position the manometer in line with your eye level.
- Palpate the brachial or radial pulse with your fingertips while inflating the cuff.
- Inflate the cuff to 30 mm Hg above the point where the pulse disappears.
- Place the bell of your stethoscope over the point where you felt the pulse, as shown in the bottom photo. Using the bell will help you better hear Korotkoff's sounds, which indicate pulse.
- Release the valve slowly and note the point at which the Korotkoff's sounds reappear. The start of the pulse sound indicates the systolic pressure.
- The sounds will become muffled and then disappear. The last Korotkoff's sound you hear is the diastolic pressure.

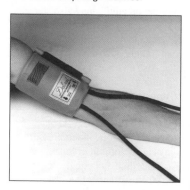

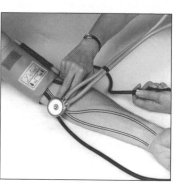

mize the number of times the patient needs to change position. By using a systematic approach, you'll also be less likely to forget an area.

No matter where you start your physical assessment, you'll use four techniques: inspection, palpation, percussion, and auscultation. The techniques are used in sequence, except when performing an abdominal assessment. Because palpation and percussion can alter bowel sounds, the sequence for assessing the abdomen is inspection, auscultation, percussion, and palpation. Let's look at each technique in the sequence, one at a time.

Inspection

Inspect the patient using seeing, smelling, and hearing to check for normal conditions and deviations. Performed correctly, inspection can reveal more

Types of palpation

The two types of palpation, light and deep, provide different types of assessment information.

Light palpation
Depress the skin ½" to ¾" (1.5 to 2 cm) with your finger pads, using the lightest touch possible. Perform light palpation to feel for surface abnormalities. Assess the area for texture, tenderness, temperature, moisture, elasticity, pulsations, superficial organs, and masses.

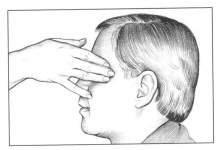

Deep palpation
Depress the skin 1½" to 2" (3.5 to 5 cm), using firm, deep pressure. If needed, use one hand on top of the other to exert firmer pressure. Deep palpation is used to feel internal organs and masses for size, shape, tenderness, symmetry, and mobility.

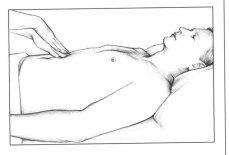

than other techniques. Proper lighting is essential.

Inspection begins when you first meet the patient and continues throughout the health history and physical examination. As you assess each body system, check for color, size, location, movement, texture, symmetry, odors, and sounds.

Palpation

Palpation consists of using different parts of your hand to touch and feel, using various degrees of pressure. Palpation is used to identify certain characteristics of the area being assessed, Fingernails should be short and hands

warm. Palpate tender areas last, and move from light to deep palpation. Tell your patient what you're palpating and why. (See *Types of palpation*.)

Don't forget to wear gloves, especially when palpating mucous membranes or other areas where you might come in contact with body fluids.

As you palpate each body system, evaluate the following features:
- texture—rough or smooth?
- temperature—warm, hot, or cold?
- moisture—dry, wet, or moist?
- motion, mobility—fixed or mobile, still or vibrating?
- consistency of structures—solid or fluid filled?

Types of percussion

Percussion technique can be characterized as direct or indirect. Direct and blunt percussion elicit tenderness; indirect percussion, sounds that give clues to the makeup of the underlying tissue.

Direct percussion
Using one or two fingers, tap directly on the body part. Ask the patient to tell you which areas are painful, and watch his face for signs of discomfort. This technique is commonly used to assess an adult patient's sinuses for tenderness.

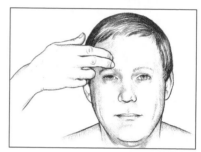

Blunt percussion
Blunt percussion is used to detect tenderness over organs such as kidneys by placing one hand flat on the body surface and using the fist of the other hand to strike the back of the hand flat on the body surface.

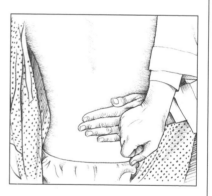

Indirect percussion
Press the distal part of the middle finger of your nondominant hand firmly on the body part. Keep the rest of your hand off the body surface. Flex the wrist, but not the forearm, of your dominant hand. Using the middle finger of your dominant hand, tap quickly and directly over the point where your nondominant middle finger touches the patient's skin, keeping the fingers perpendicular. Listen to the sounds produced.

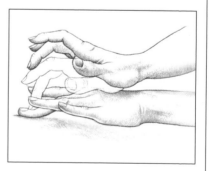

Percussion sounds and their sources

Percussion produces different sounds, depending on the underlying body structure. This chart offers a quick guide to these sounds and their sources.

Sound	Quality of sound	Where it's heard	Source
Tympany	Drumlike	Over enclosed air	Puffed-out cheek; air in bowel
Resonance	Hollow	Over areas of part air and part solid	Normal lung
Hyperresonance	Booming	Over air	Lung with emphysema
Dullness	Thudlike	Over solid tissue	Spleen, heart, liver, full bladder
Flatness	Flat	Over dense tissue	Muscle, bone

- size and shape
- tenderness.

Percussion

Percussion involves tapping your fingers or hands quickly and sharply against parts of the patient's body, usually the chest or abdomen. (See *Types of percussion*.) The technique helps you to locate organ borders, identify organ shape and position, and determine if an organ is solid or filled with fluid or gas.

Percussion requires a skilled touch and an ear trained to detect slight variations in sound. Organs and tissues produce sounds of varying loudness, pitch, and duration, depending on their density. For instance, air-filled cavities, such as the lungs, produce markedly different sounds than the liver and other dense tissues. (See *Percussion sounds and their sources*.)

As you percuss, move gradually from areas of resonance to those of dullness, and then compare sounds. Also compare sounds on one side of the body to sounds on the other side.

Auscultation

Auscultation, usually the last step, involves listening for various breath, heart, vascular, and bowel sounds with a stethoscope. To prevent the spread of infection among patients, clean the heads and end pieces with alcohol or a disinfectant. Your stethoscope should have snugly fitting ear plugs, which you'll position toward your nose; tubing no longer than 15″ (38 cm), with an internal diameter not greater than ⅛″ (0.3 cm); a diaphragm; and a bell.

HOW TO AUSCULTATE

Hold the diaphragm firmly against the patient's skin, enough to leave a slight ring afterward. Hold the bell lightly against his skin, enough to form a seal. (Holding the bell too firmly causes the skin to act as a diaphragm, obliterating low-pitched sounds.)

Hair on the patient's chest may cause friction on the end piece, which can mimic abnormal breath sounds such as crackles. You can minimize this problem by lightly dampening the hair before auscultating.

Also, keep these points in mind:
- Provide a quiet environment.
- Make sure the area to be auscultated is exposed. Don't try to auscultate over a gown or bed linens because they can interfere with sounds.
- Warm the stethoscope head in your hand.
- Close your eyes to help focus your attention.
- Listen to and try to identify the characteristics of one sound at a time.

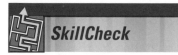

SkillCheck

1. You obtain subjective information by:
   a. observing the patient.
   b. performing a physical assessment.
   c. checking laboratory reports.
   d. listening to the patient's descriptions of his symptoms.

Answer: d. Subjective information is gathered solely from the patient's account.

2. Why shouldn't you palpate both carotid arteries at the same time?
   a. You can't assess the pulse accurately unless you palpate the arteries one at a time.
   b. You may cause transient hypertension.
   c. You'll impair cerebral blood flow and function.
   d. You may cause severe tachycardia.

Answer: c. Putting pressure on both sides of the patient's neck will obstruct the flow of blood to the brain, affecting neurologic functioning.

3. Which sequence should you follow when assessing the abdomen?
   a. Inspection, percussion, auscultation, palpation
   b. Auscultation, inspection, percussion, palpation
   c. Inspection, auscultation, percussion, palpation
   d. Auscultation, inspection, palpation, percussion

Answer: c. Because percussion and palpation can alter bowel sounds, they should be done at the end. Thus, the proper sequence is inspection, auscultation, percussion, and palpation.

4. In a cardiovascular emergency, which arteries should you palpate to assess the patient's pulse?
   a. Radial and brachial arteries
   b. Brachial and femoral arteries
   c. Carotid and radial arteries
   d. Carotid and femoral arteries

Answer: d. The carotid and femoral arteries should be used because they're larger and closer to the heart, and they more accurately reflect the heart's activity.

5. Your patient is experiencing abdominal pain in the right upper quadrant. Which area of the abdomen should you palpate last?

    a. Left upper quadrant
    b. Right upper quadrant
    c. Left lower quadrant
    d. Right lower quadrant

Answer: b. Because you should always palpate tender areas last, avoid doing the right upper quadrant until after you do the others.

Focusing the 3-minute assessment

The 3-minute assessment isn't a new concept. After all, rapid, focused assessments are routine for nurses in such places as critical care units and emergency departments. But today, you need rapid assessment skills no matter where you work. That's because the typical patient is now more acutely ill than ever, and most nurses are busier than ever.

When you or your patient first notice a change in his condition, you need pertinent information in a hurry. To obtain it, your assessment must be quick and systematic. That's exactly what this chapter gives you—guidelines for a rapid systematic approach to exploring various system-specific symptoms, based on the history and physical assessment techniques presented in chapter 1, Basic assessment review. This chapter highlights assessment techniques specific to the body system or complaint of the patient.

Components of the 3-minute assessment

You won't always want or need to assess a patient in 3 minutes. However, rapid assessment is crucial when you must intervene quickly, such as when a hospitalized patient complains of a change in physical, mental, or emotional status.

You may also perform a rapid assessment to confirm a diagnostic finding. For example, if arterial blood gas analysis indicates a low oxygen content, you'll quickly assess the patient for other signs of oxygen deprivation, such as an increased respiratory rate and cyanosis.

GENERAL GUIDELINES

Assess the patient quickly and systematically. To save time, cover some of the assessment components simultaneously. For example, make your general observations while checking the patient's vital signs or asking history questions.

Be flexible. You won't necessarily use the same sequence each time. Let the patient's chief complaint and your initial observations guide your assessment. Sometimes, you may be unable to obtain a quick history and, instead, will have to rely on your observations and the information in the patient's chart.

Keep the patient calm and cooperative. If you don't know him, first introduce yourself by name and title. Remain calm, and reassure him that you can help. If your demeanor can reduce his anxiety, he'll be more likely to give you accurate information.

Avoid drawing quick conclusions. In particular, don't assume that the patient's chief complaint is related to the admitting diagnosis.

When every minute counts, follow these steps.

Assess airway, breathing, and circulation (ABCs)

Although assessing airway, breathing, and circulation is your first priority, the assessment may just require a momentary observation. However, if the patient is unconscious or having difficulty breathing, assess him more thoroughly to detect the problem and intervene immediately. (See *Adult emergency care interventions,* pages 24 and 25.)

Make general observations

Note the patient's mental status, general appearance, and level of consciousness (LOC) for clues to the nature and severity of his condition.

Assess vital signs

The seriousness and urgency of the patient's chief complaint and your general observation of his condition will determine how extensively you measure his vital signs initially. Take the patient's body temperature, pulse, respiratory rate, and blood pressure, and ask about pain. Many facilities include pain as the "fifth" vital sign. These results provide a quick overview of physiologic condition as well as valuable information about the heart, lungs, and blood vessels.

Conduct the health history

Use pointed questions to explore the patient's perception of his chief complaint. Find out what's bothering him the most. Ask him to quantify the problem. Does he, for instance, feel worse today than he did yesterday? Such questions will help you focus your assessment. If time does not permit or the patient can't respond, obtain information from other sources, such as family members, medical history, admission forms, and the patient's chart.

Perform the physical assessment

First, concentrate on areas related to the patient's chief complaint—the abdomen, for example, if the patient complains of abdominal pain. Compare the results with baseline data, if available.

Sometimes, you may have to perform a complete head-to-toe or body systems assessment—for instance, if a patient is unresponsive (yet has no breathing or circulatory problems) or is confused and, thus, unreliable. However, in most cases, the patient's chief complaint, your general observations, and your findings regarding the patient's vital signs will guide your assessment.

PEDIATRIC AND ELDERLY PATIENTS

When you perform a rapid assessment on a child or an elderly patient, you'll need to modify your approach. The following sections cover the key differences you should be aware of when assessing these patients.

Assessing pediatric patients

You may find rapid assessment a particular challenge with an infant or child. Look for nonverbal cues. Consider communication difficulties, for example. A child who hasn't yet mastered language skills can't describe the
(Text continues on page 26.)

Adult emergency care interventions

This chart reflects current American Heart Association recommendations and outlines the steps you'll take after you determine that your patient is in distress.

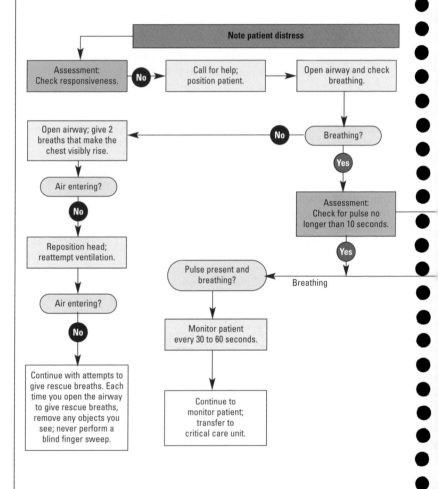

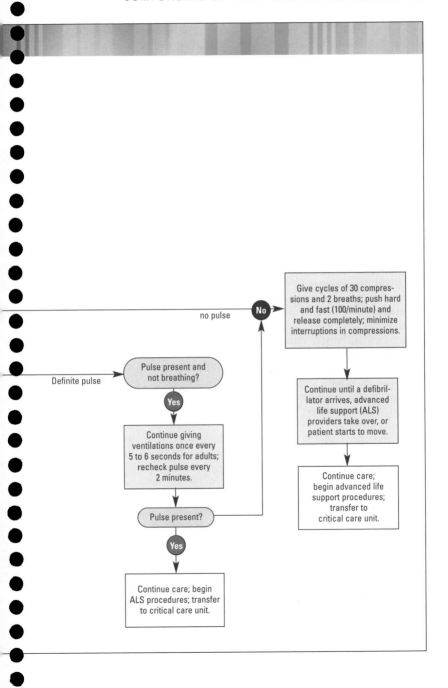

problem in detail, if at all. So you must be alert for behavior that points to a problem, such as crying, irritability, restlessness, and lethargy. Then let the child's behavior help guide your assessment. If the child is lethargic, for instance, you'll need to assess LOC. If he is having pain, observe for signs and use a pediatric assessment tool quantify.

As when assessing any patient, communicate control and friendliness. Be gentle and considerate and be positive and direct in all communications. Identify yourself clearly, and speak in terms that the child can understand. Above all, be honest when describing procedures; failure to prepare the child for a potentially frightening or painful procedure may destroy his sense of trust in you and other health care providers, interfering with your ability to perform assessments and provide care.

Because a child's normal separation anxiety is heightened in an acute situation, allow the parents to remain in the room during your assessment, if possible. Allowing them to stay with the child may help ease anxiety and increase cooperativeness.

When you examine an infant or young child, sequence your assessment techniques to inspect, auscultate, palpate, and percuss. Because other assessment procedures may make the child cry, auscultate right after inspection.

GENERAL OBSERVATIONS

You'll make your general observations in basically the same way you would with an adult. Focus on LOC, affect, behavioral and verbal responses, skin condition, posture, activity level, motor coordination, language, maturity level, and ability to understand and cooperate with the assessment.

Consider that a child may be more spontaneous and restless than an adult. He may stare, ask questions with unabashed curiosity, and readily express emotion.

Observe the patient for signs of anxiety, including thumb sucking, nail biting, and rocking. If a parent is present, observe the parent-child interaction.

Note the child's mental status. A sick infant may be irritable or lethargic, whereas a toddler may sulk or scream. An older child who is sick may be tearful, withdrawn, or irritable. Ask his parents how his behavior differs from normal. Unusual behavior tells you something is wrong.

VITAL SIGNS

The normal ranges for vital signs vary with age. In general, the younger the child, the higher the pulse and respiratory rates. (See *Normal pediatric vital signs*.) Normal blood pressure values vary with age, sex, and height.

Temperature. Temperature is more labile in infants and young children than in older children and adults. What's more, the degree of fever doesn't always correlate with the severity of the illness. For example, an infant with a severe infection may have a normal or even subnormal temperature, whereas a young child with a minor infection may have a high temperature.

When assessing a child with a febrile illness, keep in mind that you may detect a 10% increase in pulse and respirations for each degree centigrade of temperature increase.

Normal pediatric vital signs

In children, normal pulse rates and respiratory rates vary with age, as shown in the chart below.

Age	Pulse rate (beats/minute)	Respiratory rate (breaths/minute)
Neonate (1 to 28 days)	90 to 180	30 to 60
1 to 6 months	80 to 180	20 to 40
6 to 12 months	75 to 155	20 to 40
1 to 2 years	70 to 150	20 to 40
2 to 6 years	68 to 138	20 to 40
6 to 10 years	65 to 125	15 to 25
10 to 14 years	55 to 115	15 to 25

Pulse. You can feel a carotid pulse in an older child, but you may not be able to find it in an infant because his neck is too short. Auscultate the infant's apical pulse, or palpate his brachial pulse and count for a full 60 seconds.

Note any increase, decrease, or irregularity, remembering that heart rate in infants and children is labile and more sensitive to stressful events. A bounding pulse may indicate a large left-to-right shunt produced by a patent ductus arteriosus. A weak, thready pulse may indicate diminished cardiac output or the presence of peripheral vasoconstriction.

Children may normally have sinus arrhythmia, in which the heart rate increases with inspiration and decreases with expiration. If your patient can cooperate, ask him to hold his breath for a few seconds—his heart rate will become regular if he has sinus arrhythmia but will continue to be irregular if he has a true arrhythmia. Keep in mind that tachycardia is a common response to such stressors as anxiety, fever, hypoxia, hypercapnia, and hypovolemia. Note any bradycardia (age specific). Even though it may be asymptomatic, bradycardia is a late ominous sign in pediatric patients.

Respirations. In infants and young children, breathing is primarily diaphragmatic and thoracic excursion is minimal. As a result, you may find it easier to obtain the respiratory rate by observing abdominal rather than thoracic excursion. Also, an infant's respiratory rates change every 15 to 30 seconds. To obtain an accurate count, try to assess an infant's respiratory rate for a full 60 seconds. You also need to be aware that a child's respiratory rate is more responsive than an adult's to illness, emotion, and exercise. In fact, with stress the rate can double.

A pediatric patient's respiratory rate can provide valuable clues to life-threatening conditions. Quiet tachypnea—rapid respirations without signs of respiratory distress—can alert you to such problems as metabolic acidosis. Quiet tachypnea results from the body attempting to maintain normal pH by increasing minute ventilation; this causes a compensatory respiratory alkalosis.

Acutely ill infants and children with slow respiratory rates require careful assessment. A decreasing respiratory rate is an ominous trend in such conditions as hypothermia and central nervous system depression. However, such a decrease may just indicate fatigue—especially in a patient whose respiratory rate was previously elevated. Respiratory depression is the number one reason for bradycardia in pediatric patients. Identify structural abnormalities of the thoracic area during your assessment. Also check respiratory effort for abnormalities, such as retractions or nasal flaring.

Blood pressure. Many facilities now use electronic blood pressure machines to assess blood pressure in infants; however, children are usually able and willing to cooperate when a stethoscope and sphygmomanometer are used. Whether measuring blood pressure electronically or manually, remember to choose the appropriate cuff size; inappropriate cuff size can affect the accuracy of your results. Blood pressure measurements are routinely performed for children age 2 and older,

or for any child, regardless of age, whose history or physical assessment findings deem it necessary.

Because children have a proportionately smaller blood volume, even seemingly minor injuries can produce significant blood loss, possibly leading to shock. Because shock can develop insidiously, careful monitoring and frequent assessments are necessary. *Keep in mind that hypotension is a late and commonly sudden sign of shock.* A fall of even 10 mm Hg in systolic blood pressure warrants close observation.

HEALTH HISTORY

During the health history interview, direct as many questions as possible to the child. Of course, with a young child, you'll have to rely on the parents to provide most of the information. But even a young child can discuss symptoms to some degree and confirm the information the parents give you.

After asking about the chief complaint, explore pertinent medical history. Possible topics include prenatal history and birth complications, congenital abnormalities, neonatal complications, developmental history, nutritional status, childhood illnesses, and immunizations.

Assessing geriatric patients

When assessing an elderly patient, use the same techniques you use for other adults. However, you need to take into account the physiologic and biological changes that are a normal part of aging. Impaired respiratory and cardiovascular functions may make your patient more susceptible to airway, breathing, and circulation difficulties. Decreased function in other body systems may exacerbate the patient's current condition. An elderly patient may also have one or more chronic diseases, and polypharmacy may potentially present problems in the elderly patient.

Even though you need to consider age-related changes when assessing an elderly patient, avoid stereotypical misconceptions because they can interfere with an accurate assessment. For example, not all elderly patients are frail, slow-moving, and sensory impaired.

During your assessment, follow these guidelines:

■ Stand or sit where the patient can see you as you speak to him.
■ Be aware of common age-related vision difficulties.
■ Speak clearly, distinctly, and slowly, in a well-modulated voice.

GENERAL OBSERVATIONS

An elderly patient may have several chronic health problems involving more than one system that can complicate the disorder underlying his chief complaint. An elderly patient's symptoms may also be nonspecific. For example, a patient who has an acute systemic infection or a stroke may show only one symptom—confusion. Because the brain is the most vulnerable organ in elderly patients, any new illness or physical problem is likely to cause a change in mental status. These changes can include confusion, agitation and, perhaps, delirium. Look for an underlying problem in any patient with mental status changes.

When you assess your patient, also remember that he may have decreased function in all body systems. Expect him to have slowed intestinal motility, diminished renal function, decreased

sensation and reflexes, reduced muscle mass, and weakened bones and joints. A hip or pelvic fracture, for instance, may result from just a small amount of force. Elderly patients metabolize medications at a slower rate.

VITAL SIGNS

An elderly patient is likely to have reduced cardiac output (by as much as 35% in those older than age 70), decreased arterial wall elasticity, and arterial and venous insufficiency. Such factors make an elderly patient more likely than a younger one to have chronic heart disease, hypertension, and atherosclerosis.

Pulse. The patient's peripheral pulses may be decreased if he has chronic venous and arterial insufficiency. Weak or absent peripheral pulses don't necessarily indicate shock or circulatory impairment in such a patient.

Respirations. When assessing the patient's respirations, expect chest expansion to be decreased because of muscle weakness, general physical disability, a sedentary lifestyle, and possible calcifications of the rib articulations.

Blood pressure. To ensure an accurate reading, measure blood pressure in both arms. Evaluate the patient's pulse and blood pressure against what's normal for him. Because of increased vagal tone, an elderly patient may have a slower heart rate, although in some cases the heart rate becomes more rapid with age. Ectopic beats, fairly common in elderly patients, may produce irregularities in heart rhythm. If your patient has a sclerosed aorta, you may note an elevated systolic blood pressure with a normal diastolic pressure.

Pain. Elderly patients may be vague when describing complaints of pain. Some may be stoic and attempt to tolerate pain, which may be an indicator of a more serious problem. Delays in reporting pain may cause a change in their vital signs (tachycardia, tachypnea, hypertension) and a change in LOC. Elderly patients are also more sensitive to the effects of pain medications.

HEALTH HISTORY

Help the patient focus on the most important aspects of his history. He'll probably have an extensive medical history—and difficulty relating it chronologically. Help him by asking questions that keep him on track. For example, you might ask if he had a particular illness, injury, or operation before or after his last birthday. Remember to keep your language simple and direct.

If the patient's cognitive or sensory function is diminished, modify your health history interview. Otherwise, focus on the same areas you would for any adult—but place special emphasis on medication use.

When exploring the patient's chief complaint, remember that pain tolerance may be increased or pain sensations diminished from sensory loss. Don't underestimate the severity of the problem just because he doesn't report severe pain.

Be aware that your patient may hesitate to report symptoms because he attributes them to "old age" and feels that nothing can be done to ease them. The patient also may have adjusted to gradual changes and simply may not have noticed the symptoms.

EXPLORING SYMPTOMS

A clear understanding of your patient's symptoms is essential for guiding your 3-minute assessment. As you and your patient explore the symptoms, you'll form a first impression as to how you need to respond. If a symptom is acute and severe, you may need to perform a physical assessment immediately. If the symptom seems mild to moderate, you may be able to take a more complete history. (See *Evaluating a symptom.*)

One method of gaining an understanding of your patient's symptoms involves using the mnemonic device PQRST as a guide.

Provocative or palliative

Your questions to the patient should be aimed at finding out what causes the symptom and what makes it better or worse. The following are questions that may help you elicit this information.
- What were you doing when you first noticed it?
- What seems to trigger it? Stress? Position? Certain activities? An argument? (For a physical sign such as eye discharge: What seems to cause it or make it worse? For a psychological symptom such as depression: Does the depression occur after specific events?)
- What relieves the symptom? Changing diet? Changing position? Taking medication? Being active?
- What makes the symptom worse?

Quality or quantity

Try to find out how the symptom feels, looks, or sounds. Also, have the patient tell you how much of the symptom he's experiencing. The following questions may help the patient express this to you.

Evaluating a symptom

Your patient may be vague in describing his chief complaint. Using your interviewing skills, you may discover his problem is related to abdominal distention. Now what? This flowchart will help you decide what to do next, using abdominal distention as the patient's chief complaint.

Question the patient to identify what's bothering him physically.
He tells you, "My stomach gets bloated."

⬇

Form a first impression. Does the patient's condition alert you to an emergency? For example, does he say the bloating developed suddenly? Does he mention that other signs or symptoms occur with it, such as sweating or light-headedness? (Both are indicators of hypovolemia.)

YES | **NO**

Take a brief history to gather more clues. For example, ask the patient if he has severe abdominal pain or difficulty breathing or if he ever had an abdominal injury.

Now, take a thorough history to get an overview of the patient's condition. Ask him about associated signs or symptoms. Note especially GI disorders that can lead to abdominal distention.

⬇ ⬇

Perform a focused physical examination to quickly determine the severity of the patient's condition. Check for bruising, lacerations, changes in bowel sounds, or abdominal rigidity.

Now, thoroughly examine the patient to evaluate the chief sign or symptom and to detect additional signs and symptoms. Place the patient in a recumbent position, and observe him for abdominal asymmetry. Inspect the skin, auscultate for bowel sounds, percuss and palpate the abdomen, and measure his abdominal girth.

⬇ ⬇

Evaluate your findings. Are emergency signs or symptoms present, such as abdominal rigidity or abnormal bowel sounds?

YES | **NO**

Based on your findings, intervene appropriately to stabilize the patient's condition. Notify the doctor immediately, place the patient in a supine position, administer oxygen, and start an I.V. line. GI or nasogastric tube insertion and emergency surgery may be needed.

Review your findings to consider possible causes, such as cancer, bladder distention, cirrhosis, heart failure, or gastric dilation.

⬇ ⬇

After the patient's condition is stabilized, review your findings to consider possible causes, such as trauma, large-bowel obstruction, mesenteric artery occlusion, or peritonitis.

Evaluate your findings and devise an appropriate care plan. Position the patient comfortably, administer analgesics, and prepare the patient for diagnostic tests.

■ How would you describe the symptom—that is, how does it feel, look, or sound?

■ How much are you experiencing now? Is it so much that it prevents you from performing certain activities? Is it more or less than you experienced at any other time?

Region or radiation

It's important to pinpoint the location of the patient's symptom. Besides asking the following questions, have the patient point to the exact locations on his body where he's experiencing the symptom and to any areas to which it spreads.

■ Where does the symptom occur?

■ In the case of pain, does it travel down your back or arms, up your neck, or down your legs?

Severity

The acuity of a symptom will impact the timeliness of further assessments. Having the patient rate the symptom on a scale of 1 to 10, with 10 being most severe, can help you determine how quickly you need to proceed to a physical assessment. The following questions will also give you clues to the severity of a symptom.

■ How bad is the symptom at its worst? Does it force you to lie down, sit down, or slow down?

■ Does the symptom seem to be getting better, getting worse, or staying about the same?

Timing

Determine when the symptom began and how it began, whether gradually or suddenly. If the symptom is intermittent, find out how often it occurs.

■ On what date and time did the symptom first occur?

■ How did the symptom start? Suddenly? Gradually?

■ How often do you experience the symptom? Hourly? Daily? Weekly? Monthly?

■ When do you usually experience the symptom? During the day? At night? In the early morning? Does it awaken you? Does it occur before, during, or after meals? Does it occur seasonally?

■ How long does an episode of the symptom last?

Pain assessment

The sensation of pain alerts us to injury or illness and serves as a protective mechanism. Pain is complex and can be challenging to understand and treat. Your focused assessment of pain can provide valuable information toward the diagnosis and treatment plan for the patient.

Check the patient for pain during your history and physical assessment. The Joint Commission on Accreditation of Healthcare Organizations has implemented standards for the management of pain to make sure patients receive effective pain relief. Levels of pain experienced are influenced by physical pathology, cultural and social factors, expectations, mood, and perceptions of control. Patients have dramatically different pain thresholds and tolerances and ways of expressing pain. Even if you think the patient's behavior doesn't match his report of pain, remember the first principle of pain management: Pain is whatever the patient

Differentiating acute and chronic pain

Acute pain may cause certain physiologic and behavioral changes that you won't observe in a patient with chronic pain.

Type of pain	Physiologic evidence	Behavioral evidence
Acute	• Increased respirations • Increased pulse • Increased blood pressure • Dilated pupils • Diaphoresis	• Restlessness • Distraction • Worry • Distress
Chronic	• Normal respirations • Normal pulse • Normal blood pressure • Normal pupil size • No diaphoresis	• Reduced or absent physical activity • Despair, depression • Hopelessness

says it is, occurring whenever he says it does. His self-report of the presence and severity of pain is the most accurate, reliable means of pain assessment.

When a patient reports pain, it's important to promptly assess and implement actions to treat or manage the pain. Your focused assessment should differentiate between acute and chronic pain. (See *Differentiating acute and chronic pain*.) Acute pain may be a symptom of an underlying problem and a more detailed assessment of the pain may yield information leading to a diagnosis and formulation of an appropriate plan.

Many pain scales are available to quantify pain intensity—one of pain's most subjective aspects. These provide a consistent measurement of pain for your patient. The numerical rating scale is the most commonly used pain rating scale. Ask the patient to rate his pain on a scale from 0 to 10 with 0 representing no pain and 10 representing

the worst pain imaginable. Although it's the easiest, it may be too abstract for some patients and isn't appropriate for children. When you assess a patient for pain, consider the following aspects of pain:
- location
- type—acute or chronic
- onset and duration
- quantity (intensity, severity)
- quality (such as burning, stabbing, cramping, soreness)
- relief measures
- aggravating factors
- time it occurs

Observation of the patient with pain can be useful for comparison, evaluation, and follow-up treatment. Certain behaviors are associated with patients in pain. (See *Pain behavior checklist,* page 34.)

CHECKLIST

Pain behavior checklist

A pain behavior is something a patient uses to communicate pain, distress, or suffering. Place a check in the box next to each behavior you observe or infer while talking with your patient.

- ❏ Grimacing
- ❏ Moaning
- ❏ Sighing
- ❏ Clenching teeth
- ❏ Holding or supporting the painful body area
- ❏ Sitting rigidly
- ❏ Frequently shifting posture or position
- ❏ Moving in a guarded or protective manner
- ❏ Moving very slowly
- ❏ Limping
- ❏ Taking medication
- ❏ Using a cane, cervical collar, or other prosthetic device
- ❏ Walking with an abnormal gait
- ❏ Requesting help with walking
- ❏ Stopping frequently while walking
- ❏ Lying down during the day
- ❏ Avoiding physical activity
- ❏ Being irritable
- ❏ Asking such questions as, "Why did this happen to me?"
- ❏ Asking to be relieved from tasks or activities

DOCUMENTING YOUR 3-MINUTE ASSESSMENT

After you've completed your 3-minute assessment, you need to document your findings, interventions, and the patient's response. Identify known baseline values and compare them with current values. This will help you identify, define, and analyze the patient's problem. You'll establish priorities for treatment based on the findings.

Be accurate, concise, and current. Organize your information so other members of the health care team can easily follow it. Try to document as soon as you finish, using only accepted abbreviations and specific words. When documenting changes in the patient's condition, avoid being subjective and focus on the facts only when there is a behavior change. Keep in mind:

- immediate general observations
- vital signs
- history of chief complaint
- exact words of patient or source of information
- your inspection, palpation, percussion, and auscultation findings
- use of anatomic landmarks.

SkillCheck

1. What should be your first step in a 3-minute assessment?
   a. Taking the patient's history
   b. Performing a physical assessment based on his symptom
   c. Taking the patient's temperature
   d. Assessing the patient's airway, breathing, and circulation

Answer: d. Assessing airway, breathing, and circulation may take only seconds of your time. It will direct the rest of your rapid assessment in that you may need to stop and intervene immediately.

2. What *isn't* a guideline for performing a 3-minute assessment?
   a. Perform the 3-minute assessment the same way every time.
   b. Assess the patient not only quickly but systematically.
   c. If you don't already know the patient, introduce yourself, then as you perform the assessment, remain calm and keep the patient calm.
   d. Avoid drawing conclusions.

Answer: a. Try to be flexible in your approach. Let the patient's chief complaint and your initial observations guide your assessment.

3. The mnemonic device PQRST stands for:
   a. practices, quantity, region, source, and tone.
   b. provoking or palliative factors, quality or quantity, region or radiation, severity, and timing.
   c. provoking factors, quality or quantity, region or radiation, source, and tone.
   d. practices, quantity, region, severity, and time.

Answer: b. These factors combined will give you a clear understanding of your patient's symptoms.

4. When auscultating your pediatric patient, you notice that his heart rate increases with inspiration and decreases with expiration. You note that his heart rate becomes regular when you auscultate while he's holding his breath. This is:
   a. a normal finding.
   b. an abnormal finding.

Answer: a. A true arrhythmia is present even while the patient holds his breath. This child has a normal sinus arrhythmia.

5. What factor *shouldn't* be considered when assessing an elderly patient?
   a. An elderly patient may have one or more chronic diseases.
   b. A new illness or physical problem is likely to cause a change in mental status because in elderly patients the brain is the most vulnerable organ.
   c. Most elderly patients have trouble hearing, so you'll need to speak loudly when obtaining the health history.
   d. The elderly patient may have slowed intestinal motility and weakened bones and joints.

Answer: c. Avoid stereotypical misconceptions when working with patients. Although you should always speak clearly and distinctly when assessing a patient, it isn't always necessary to raise your voice when assessing an elderly patient.

Documentation

Documentation or charting is the process of keeping a complete record of a patient's care. Documentation is vital for communication in health care. Decisions, actions, and changes related to the patient's care are often based on the documentation. Nurses must have the skills to produce an accurate, effective, and efficient record of care. It's important that nurses document patient information in a clear, concise, organized manner.

Nursing documentation communicates to other members of the health care team the nurse's contribution to the diagnosis, treatment, and care of the patient. It provides a complete, accurate, legible record, which must be easily retrievable and readable. Documentation is part of the nurse's routine; it should clearly illustrate the assessment—the first step in the nursing process. It's important to document your initial assessment, interventions, and reassessment as you care for your patient.

A patient's medical record may be read by a wide audience including:
- other members of the health care team
- performance improvement monitors
- reviewers from accrediting, certifying, and licensing organizations
- peer reviewers
- Medicare agents and insurance company reviewers

- researchers and teachers
- attorneys and judges.

Accuracy

Accurate nursing documentation is important for many reasons including:
- professional responsibility and accountability
- communication
- health care evaluation
- legal protection
- research and education
- accreditation and licensure
- reimbursement from insurance companies
- performance improvement
- compliance with nurse practice acts.

PROFESSIONAL ACCOUNTABILITY AND COMPLIANCE
Accurate nursing documentation shows that you have met your responsibilities to the patient and establishes compliance with the documentation requirements of your health care facility, professional organizations, and state law.

COMMUNICATION
The medical record is the main source of information for all health care providers who see the same patient. Even though nurses are considered care

managers and document the most information, a complete picture of the patient's care is presented through multidisciplinary health care notes.

HEALTH CARE EVALUATION

Reviewers, insurance companies, Medicare agents, lawyers, and judges all evaluate health care, and documentation is one way to prove that you're providing high-quality care. It's also a record of the patient's responses to care and any changes you make in his care plan.

LEGAL PROTECTION

Accurate and thorough documentation shows that the care provided meets the patient's needs and wishes, and that you're following accepted standards of nursing care mandated by law, your profession, and your health care facility. Proper documentation communicates crucial clinical information to caregivers so they make fewer errors. It can determine whether you or your employer wins or loses a legal dispute. Medical records are used as evidence in cases involving disability, personal injury, and mental competency. Poor documentation is the main issue in many malpractice cases.

RESEARCH AND EDUCATION

In accordance with the Health Insurance Portability and Accountability Act regulations, researchers and nurse educators may study medical records to determine the effectiveness of care. They may identify ways to improve documentation (revise current forms, create more efficient forms). The need for simple, accurate point-of-care documentation encourages researchers to develop new technologies to improve

communication between health care providers, improve patient safety, and optimize a nurse's time. Records are also reviewed for patient education and compliance with treatment regimens.

ACCREDITATION AND LICENSURE

For a facility to remain accredited, caregivers must document care that reflects the care standards set by national organizations such as the American Nurses Association and the Joint Commission on Accreditation of Healthcare Organizations (JCAHO). Licensed organizations are required to establish policies and procedures for operation; substandard documentation may jeopardize accreditation and licensure.

REIMBURSEMENT

Reimbursement from Medicare and insurance companies depends heavily on accurate nursing documentation, which provides justification for reimbursement. Most insurance companies base reimbursement for skilled medical and nursing care on necessity only. Payment for patient care may be denied if the nurse's charting doesn't support that the care (such as home care visits) was necessary.

PERFORMANCE IMPROVEMENT

States and JCAHO require health care facilities to monitor, evaluate, and seek ways to improve the quality of care for their patients. Hospital risk managers and accreditation agencies use nursing documentation to evaluate the quality of patient care. Additionally, each facility has a multidisciplinary performance improvement committee that often bases its recommendations on the medical records.

NURSE PRACTICE ACTS

Nurse practice acts are state laws that spell out what duties nurses can perform in that state. State nurse practice acts are revised frequently and when they change, charting requirements usually change as well. You must be especially meticulous about charting to show compliance with standards.

Documentation systems

Continuous quality improvement programs monitor and evaluate the contents of a patient's medical record and systems may need to be modified or replaced to meet your facility's needs. Know which documentation systems are acceptable in your facility. Although formats for documentation vary between settings, the content shouldn't. For consistency and thoroughness, follow the documentation standards of JCAHO and your facility's policy.

TRADITIONAL NARRATIVE CHARTING

This is a straightforward chronologic account of the patient's status, the nursing interventions performed, and the patient's responses. Flow sheets supplement the documentation included in the progress notes.

Document patient assessments as often as your facility requires and more frequently when the patient's condition changes or a new symptom develops. Organize your notes using a head-to-toe approach as you assess the patient. Be specific and document chronologically, recording exact times as you perform your targeted assessment, interventions, and responses.

PROBLEM-ORIENTED MEDICAL RECORD

The problem-oriented medical record, or POMR, focuses on specific patient problems and may be an appropriate choice for a targeted 3-minute assessment. There are five components:

■ Database—subjective and objective data about the patient form the initial care plan. Collect these data during the initial assessment and include information such as the reason for hospitalization, medications, medical history, allergies, physical and psychosocial findings, self-care abilities, educational needs, pain assessment, and discharge planning concerns.

■ Problem list—a numbered, chronologic list of the patient's problems to provide an overview of the patient's health status. Refer to the problem by number when writing your notes. As problems are resolved, note the date and time, and sign or initial the record according to your facility's policy.

■ Initial plan—expected outcomes and plans for further data collection, patient care, and teaching.

■ Progress notes—typically, a note for each current problem every 24 hours or when the patient's condition changes. SOAP, SOAPIE, or SOAPIER is used to structure progress notes.

  – **S**ubjective data—the reason for seeking care
  – **O**bjective data—those that are both factual and measurable
  – **A**ssessment data—conclusions based on subjective and objective data and formulated as patient problems or nursing diagnoses
  – **P**lan—strategies for relieving the

patient's problems, which should include both short-term and long-term actions
- **I**nterventions—measures implemented to achieve expected outcomes
- **E**valuation—analysis of the effectiveness of interventions implemented
- **R**evision—changes from the original plan of care

■ Discharge summary—covers each problem on the list and notes if it was resolved. Unresolved problems must be discussed and a plan specified. Record communications with other facilities, home health agencies, and the patient.

PROBLEM-INTERVENTION-EVALUATION SYSTEM

The problem-intervention-evaluation, or PIE, system organizes information according to the patient's problems. Major categories such as respiration or pain are included on the daily assessment flow sheet and progress notes. Times of treatments and continued assessment of a specific area are tracked.

■ **P**roblem—Use data collected from your assessment to identify pertinent nursing diagnoses. Document each problem using a number system (such as P#l).

■ **I**ntervention—Document the nursing actions you take for each problem.

■ **E**valuation—Document the patient's response to interventions. Label the evaluation with an "E" followed by the problem number (such as EP#l).

FOCUS CHARTING

FOCUS charting is organized into patient-centered topics, or foci, and uses assessment data to evaluate these concerns. Documentation is done on a progress sheet with columns for the date, time, focus, and progress note. In the focus column, write the focus (as a sign or symptom) and in the progress notes column, organize information using three categories: data, action, and response (DAR). In the data category include subjective and objective information that describes the focus. In the action category, include immediate and future nursing actions based on your assessment of the patient's condition and any changes to the care plan based on your evaluation. In the response category, describe the patient's response to nursing or medical care.

CHARTING BY EXCEPTION

This system departs from traditional systems by requiring documentation of only significant or abnormal findings in the narrative portion of the record. To chart effectively, adhere to established guidelines for nursing assessments and interventions and follow written standards of practice that identify the nurse's basic responsibilities. Document only deviations from the standards and use supplemental progress notes. This format involves the use of a nursing diagnosis-based standardized care plan and several types of flow sheets.

FACT DOCUMENTATION

This system, which incorporates many of the charting by exception principles, has four key elements: **f**low sheets, **a**ssessments with baseline parameters, **c**oncise integrated progress notes and flow sheets that document the patient's condition and responses, and **t**imely entries recorded when care is given. FACT documentation begins with a complete initial baseline assessment using standardized parameters and an assessment-action flow sheet, a frequent assessment flow sheet, and progress notes. FACT documentation records nursing assessment findings and interventions that are exceptions to the norm.

CORE CHARTING

Core charting focuses on the nursing process, the core, or most important part of the documentation. It consists of a database, care plan, flow sheets, progress notes, and discharge summary. Progress notes contain information for each problem organized in the DAR format.

OUTCOME DOCUMENTATION

This system charts the patient's condition in relation to predetermined outcomes on the care plan, focusing on desired outcomes rather than problems. The *database* includes subjective and objective data identifying the patient's problems and learning needs. The database is a foundation for ongoing evaluation. The *care plan* establishes priorities, identifies expected outcomes and nursing interventions, and documents the plan. Handwritten plans, preprinted standardized plans, clinical pathways, and patient care guidelines can be used. *Expected outcome statements* describe the desired results of nursing actions. Be specific and use outcome criteria that are measurable, and include a target date or time. Outcomes are evaluated and problems are resolved if outcomes aren't met.

COMPUTERIZED DOCUMENTATION

Facilities that use computer documentation can customize features for their particular institution. When using a computerized system, you may be prompted to enter data about the patient's medical history, status, chief complaint, and assessment. Some programs may ask specific questions about the data entered and some programs may flag entries if the data are outside of a certain range. Some programs offer clinical pathways to gather further information and guide care. Other programs may compare and track patient outcomes.

Advantages

Advantages of computerized documentation include:
- standardization of clinical information
- fast, easy storage and retrieval of information
- efficient, constant updating of information with links to diverse sources of patient information
- legible charting, which prevents potential errors that can occur when retrieving or transcribing handwritten information
- quick, efficient transmittal of request slips and patient information, that helps ensure confidentiality and prompts other health care providers to take action, such as initiate a consult, order laboratory studies, or administer drugs
- easy access to patient records through a central database.

Disadvantages

Disadvantages of computerized documentation include:
- system unavailability—either accidental or scheduled
- the need for user orientation, training, and support

■ the possibility of obtaining inaccurate or incomplete information because of the use of standardized phrases and limited vocabulary

■ the potential for compromised confidentiality if security measures are neglected or if information is left displayed on the computer screen

■ the expense of implementing a computerized system.

Maintaining confidentiality of computer records is essential. Never share your password or computer signature. There's an increasing move toward using biometrics (use of fingerprints or retinal scans) for securing access to patient records. Log off of the device you are using as soon as documentation or retrieval of data is complete. Don't allow visual access of a computer screen by unauthorized persons. Properly file or dispose of any printed documents from a computerized medical record.

Rules of charting

Following fundamental rules for charting enhances communication between all members of the health care team and ensures reimbursement for your facility.

■ Chart completely, concisely, and accurately. Write clear sentences that are to the point using simple, precise language. Identify the subject of each sentence and don't be afraid to use the word "I."

■ Record observations objectively. Record just the facts, exactly what *you* see, hear, and do. Avoid opinions and assumptions. Only chart information that's relevant to the patient's care.

■ Document information promptly. Chart as soon as possible after you make an observation or provide care, noting exact times chronologically.

■ When adding a late entry (check for a policy first), label it as such; record the date and time of the entry as well as the date and time when the entry should have been made.

■ Write legibly, using only black or blue ink. Avoid misspelled words and incorrect grammar.

■ Use approved abbreviations. Know your facility's acceptable abbreviations and JCAHO's list of unacceptable abbreviations. When you have doubts about an abbreviation, spell it out. (See *Official "do not use" list,* page 42.)

■ When you make a mistake on a chart, correct it immediately by drawing a single line through the entry and writing "mistaken entry" above or beside it, along with the date and time. Then sign your name. Never erase, cover with correction fluid, or completely cross out the entry. Changing a record in any way is illegal. Don't destroy records.

■ Sign all documents as required. Sign each entry you make in your progress notes with your first name or initial, last name, and professional licensure.

■ When charting continues from one page to the next, sign each page, and at the top of the next page, write the date, the time, and the words "continued from previous page." Never leave blank spaces; write N/A if appropriate.

Official "do not use" list

The Joint Commission on Accreditation of Healthcare Organizations has agreed upon a list of dangerous abbreviations, acronyms, and symbols. Using this list should help protect patients from the effects of miscommunication in clinical documentation.

Abbreviation	Danger	Instead use
U or u (for "unit")	Mistaken for the numbers 0 or 4 (for example, 4U seen as 40 or 4u seen as 44). Also mistaken for "cc" (for example, 4u seen as 4cc).	Write "unit."
IU (for "international unit")	Mistaken for I.V. (intravenous) or 10 (ten).	Write "international unit."
q.d. (Latin abbreviation for "every day")	Mistaken for q.i.d., especially if the period after the "q" or the tail of the "q" could be seen as an "i."	Write "daily" or "once daily."
q.o.d. (Latin abbreviation for "every other day")	Mistaken for q.d. or q.i.d. if the "I" is poorly written.	Write "every other day."
Trailing zero (such as 1.0 mg)	Decimal point may be missed (for example, 1.0 may be seen as 10).	Never write a zero by itself after a decimal point (1 mg rather than 1.0 mg).
Lack of leading zero (such as .5 mg)	Decimal point may be missed (for example, .5 may be seen as 5).	Always write a zero before a decimal point (0.5 mg rather than .5 mg).
MS or MSO_4 (morphine sulfate)	Mistaken for magnesium sulfate.	Write "morphine sulfate."
$MgSO_4$ (magnesium sulfate)	Mistaken for morphine sulfate.	Write "magnesium sulfate."

Legal implications

As a nursing professional, you assume legal accountability for your practice and complete, accurate documentation may be your best protection if you're named in a malpractice lawsuit. What you say and how you say it are very important in documentation. Keeping the patient's record free from negative, inappropriate information—potential legal complications—can be a challenge when you're writing detailed narrative notes. Here are some things to avoid when you document your patient's care and status. (See *Charting don'ts.*)

Chart defensively—apply these fundamental rules of charting:

- Stick to the facts.
- Avoid labeling.
- Be specific.
- Use neutral language.
- Eliminate bias.
- Keep the record intact.

LEGAL HAZARDS

Every day you face patient care situations that could become legal issues. Be alert for potential legal hazards and know how to chart defensively when they arise. Certain situations are known hazards and your best defense is recognizing them and knowing how to chart, what to chart, when to chart, and who should chart.

Charting don'ts

Negative language and inappropriate information don't belong in a medical record and can return to haunt you in a lawsuit. The charting mistakes below are legal land mines. Avoid them.

1. Don't record staffing problems
True, staff shortages may affect patient care or contribute to an incident. However, you shouldn't mention this in a patient's chart because it can be used as legal ammunition against you if the chart lands in court. Instead, write a confidential memo to your nurse-manager, and review your facility's policy and procedure manuals to see how you're expected to handle this situation.

2. Don't record staff conflicts
Don't chart:
• disputes with other nurses (including criticisms of their care)
• questions about a doctor's treatment

• a colleague's rude or abusive behavior.

Personality clashes aren't legitimate patient care concerns. In the event of a lawsuit, the plaintiff's lawyer will exploit conflicts among codefendants.

Instead of charting these problems, talk with your nurse-manager, or consult with the doctor directly if an order puzzles you. If another nurse writes personal accusations or charges of incompetence in a chart, talk to her about the implications of doing this. Remember, you're responsible for your actions.

(continued)

Charting don'ts (continued)

3. Don't mention incident reports

Incident reports are confidential and filed separately from the patient's chart. Document only the facts of an incident in the chart, and never write "incident report" or indicate that you filed one.

For example, write: *"Found pt lying on the floor at 1250 hours. Vital signs BP 110/70, P 82, R 20, T 98.6° F. No visible bleeding or trauma. AA Ox3, PERLA, + ROM to all extremities. Pt returned to bed with all side rails up and bed in low position. Pt. stated,"I must have been sleepwalking. Notified Dr. Gary Dietrich at 1253 hours, and he saw pt at 1300 hours."*

4. Don't use words associated with errors

Terms such as *by mistake, accidentally, somehow, unintentionally, miscalculated,* and *confusing* are bonus words to the plaintiff's attorney. Steer clear of words that suggest an error was made or a patient's safety was jeopardized. Let the facts speak for themselves.

For example, suppose you gave a patient 100 mg of Demerol instead of 50 mg. Here's how to chart this without calling undue attention to it: "Pt was given Demerol 100 mg I.M. at 1300 hours for abdominal pain VAS 7/10. Dr. Smith was notified but gave no orders. Pt's vital signs remained stable."

5. Don't name a second patient

Naming a second patient in a patient's chart violates confidentiality. Instead, write "roommate," the patient's initials, or his room and bed number.

6. Don't chart casual conversations with colleagues

Telling your nurse-manager in the elevator or restroom about a patient's deteriorating condition doesn't qualify as informing her. She's likely to forget the details or may not even realize you expect her to intervene. Before notifying someone, clearly state why you're notifying the person so she can focus on the facts and take appropriate action. Otherwise, you can't chart that you informed her.

Documenting your assessment

There are two key elements to documenting an assessment—nursing history and physical (also known as subjective and objective data). An initial assessment form is called a *nursing admission* or *admission database*. For frequent reassessments, flow charts such as a frequent vital signs sheet or an assessment flow chart may help

staff record and retrieve data. Progress notes can be used to document unusual events, responses, significant observations, or interactions. Quality not quantity is important in documentation. Follow an organized pattern for documenting your assessment findings. Organize all information for one body system before proceeding to the next.

JCAHO standards recommend that your initial assessment and documentation include evaluation of:

■ physical factors, including the examination findings from your review of

Key aspects of the physical assessment

During a physical examination, your main task is to record the patient's height, weight, and vital signs and review the major body systems. Here's a typical body system review for an adult patient.

Respiratory system
Note the rate and rhythm of respirations, and auscultate the lung fields. Inspect the lips, mucous membranes, and nail beds. Also inspect sputum, noting color, consistency, and other characteristics.

Cardiovascular system
Note the color and temperature of the extremities, and assess the peripheral pulses. Check for edema and hair loss on the extremities. Inspect the neck veins, and auscultate for heart sounds.

Neurologic system
Assess the patient's level of consciousness, noting his orientation to person, place, and time and his ability to follow commands. Also assess pupillary reactions. Check extremities for movement and sensation.

Eyes, ears, nose, and throat
Assess the patient's ability to see objects with and without corrective lenses. Assess his ability to hear spoken words clearly. Inspect the eyes and ears for discharge and the nasal mucous membranes for dryness, irritation, and blood. Observe the teeth, gums, and condition of the oral mucous membranes, and palpate the lymph nodes in the neck.

GI system
Auscultate for bowel sounds in all quadrants. Note abdominal distention or ascites. Gently palpate the abdomen for tenderness. Assess the condition of the mucous membranes around the anus.

Musculoskeletal system
Assess the range of motion of major joints. Look for swelling at the joints and for contractures, muscle atrophy, or obvious deformity. Assess muscle strength of the trunk and extremities.

Genitourinary and reproductive systems
Note any bladder distention or incontinence. If indicated, inspect the genitalia for rashes, edema, or deformity. (Inspection of the genitalia may be waived at the patient's request or if no dysfunction was reported during the interview.) If indicated, inspect the genitalia for sexual maturity. Also examine the breasts, noting any abnormalities.

Integumentary system
Note any sores, lesions, scars, pressure ulcers, rashes, bruises, or petechiae. Also note the patient's skin turgor.

the patient's major body systems (see *Key aspects of the physical assessment*)
■ psychological and social factors—fears, anxieties, concerns, support systems
■ environmental factors—the patient's home and its facilities, utilities, stairs
■ self-care capabilities—the patient's ability to perform activities of daily living
■ learning needs—the level of the patient's need for teaching support
■ discharge planning needs—home care, follow-up

Establishing priorities for patient assessment

After completion of an initial assessment, the Joint Commission on Accreditation of Healthcare Organizations requires nurses to use the gathered information in prioritizing their care decisions. To systematically set priorities, follow these steps:
• Identify the patient's problems.
• Identify the patient's risk for injury.
• Identify the patient's need for help with self-care, both in the hospital and following discharge.
• Identify the educational needs of the patient and his family members.

■ input from the patient's family and friends when appropriate—if obtaining information from others, document the nature of the relationship.

JCAHO also requires nurses to use the information to prioritize their interventions. (See *Establishing priorities for patient assessment.*)

When documenting your rapid assessment, be accurate, concise, and current. Identify baseline values and compare them to your findings to help identify, define, and analyze the patient's problem. Organize your information so that it can be easily followed by other members of the health care team. Document findings using anatomic landmarks to identify areas and document any actions or care given and the patient's response. Document your 3-minute assessment as soon as you finish it. When performing a targeted

assessment, use the PQRST mnemonic device to help assess and document your findings in detail. (See *Using the PQRST device.*)

DOCUMENTING PAIN

JCAHO requires that each patient be assessed for "pain" at each encounter with a health care professional when appropriate. These standards require that patients be asked about pain and any patient who reports pain must be assessed further by licensed personnel. Your documentation will be evidence that these standards have been met. Some states consider pain the fifth vital sign and documentation of your pain assessment must accompany the vital signs. If pain is identified, JCAHO requires that the patient receive treatment, be reassessed, and followed up at intervals that ensure adequate pain management.

Document your detailed, baseline pain assessment findings. This documentation will provide valuable information for diagnosis, further action, treatment, and follow-up. It provides a baseline for use in later comparison and evaluation of effectiveness of treatment. Your facility may have a standardized documentation form or flow sheet to use for pain management. For patients with unrelieved pain, conduct frequent assessments and charting.

Document the actions you take when pain is identified, such as notifying the physician, implementing tests, and administering pain medication. Note the patient's response to each intervention followed by reassessment for recurrence of the pain.

Using the PQRST device

Use the PQRST mnemonic device to fully explore your patient's chief complaint. When you ask the questions below, encourage him to describe his symptoms in greater detail.

Provocative or palliative
- What provokes or relieves the symptom?
- Do stress, anger, certain physical positions, or other events trigger the symptom?
- What makes the symptom worsen or subside?

Quality or quantity
- What does the symptom feel, look, or sound like?
- Are you having the symptom right now? If so, is it more or less severe than usual?
- To what degree does the symptom affect your normal activities?

Region or radiation
- Where in the body does the symptom occur?
- Does the symptom appear in other regions? If so, where?

Severity
- How severe is the symptom? How would you rate it on a scale of 1 to 10, with 10 being the most severe?
- Does the symptom seem to be diminishing, intensifying, or staying about the same?

Timing
- When did the symptom begin?
- Was the onset sudden or gradual?
- How often does the symptom occur?
- How long does the symptom last?

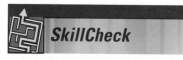

SkillCheck

1. Which statement would be correct to document when your interview with an 86-year-old, alert and oriented, male patient who lives in an adult home, raises suspicions of abuse?
  a. The patient's bruises look like they're 1 week old.
  b. The nurses at the adult home insist that the patients take a nap every afternoon.
  c. "My daughter takes my check every month and doesn't give me any money."
  d. The patient's bruises appear to be from rough treatment by the staff.

Answer: c. It's appropriate to document the patient's statement and alert the proper individuals to investigate further. Never make assumptions and document what you think about a patient situation.

2. What isn't a charting mistake?
  a. Documenting input from family members
  b. Recording of staffing issues
  c. Mentioning an incident report in your progress note
  d. Charting the name of another patient in your patient's chart

Answer: a. It's important to chart information from family members regarding a patient's care, when it's appropriate. The inclusion of staffing issues, incident reports, and other patient's names should be avoided in your documentation.

3. The medical record is the main source of information for all members of the health care team. Which would be an accurate statement?
  a. Nurse educators can't use a patient's chart for research projects.
  b. Poor documentation won't jeopardize your license as long as you follow policies and procedures.
  c. Accurate charting doesn't prove that you're providing high-quality care to your patient.
  d. Reimbursement depends on accurate documentation.

Answer: d. Insurance companies evaluate the provision of health care by chart review and reimbursement may depend on your documentation. Charts may be used for research when approved. Your license may be in jeopardy if your documentation isn't accurate because your quality of care may be questioned.

4. There are fundamental rules for charting. Which statement is accurate when incorporating these rules?
  a. Write clear sentences that are concise and accurate and include your assumptions gained from the assessment.
  b. Sign each entry in your notes with your first initial, last name, and professional licensure.
  c. Any abbreviations familiar to the staff in your facility may be used in charting.
  d. "Quality" documentation of the information you've obtained from your assessment may be documented at any point during your shift.

Answer: b. You may use your first name or initial, last name, and professional licensure when signing a chart. Assumptions should never be charted.

The Joint Commission on the Accreditation of Healthcare Organizations has issued a list of "do not use" abbreviations that must be followed, and documentation should be completed as soon as possible after you provide care or make an observation.

5. Computerized documentation is being implemented in many facilities. One of the main disadvantages of this form of charting is:
   a. the potential for compromised confidentiality.
   b. that it provides fast, easy storage and retrieval of information.
   c. that it provides legible charting, which prevents errors that can occur when transcribing orders.
   d. that it gives easy access to patient records.

Answer: a. One of the disadvantages of computerized documentation is the potential for breach of confidentiality if security measures are neglected.

Respiratory system

Of the many problems for which a patient may seek care, those involving the respiratory system pose the gravest threat to the patient. However, rapid and timely intervention can help prevent or manage serious complications.

In this chapter you'll find a review of the anatomy and physiology of the respiratory system, together with essential physical assessment techniques. The guidelines for a 3-minute assessment of symptoms related to the respiratory system are next, including general observations and vital signs pertaining to all and specific history and physical assessment techniques for each symptom.

Anatomy and physiology

The respiratory system includes the airway, lungs, bony thorax, respiratory muscles, and central nervous system. (See *Structures of the respiratory system.*) They work together to deliver oxygen to the bloodstream and remove excess carbon dioxide from the body. Knowing the basic structures and functions of the respiratory system will help you perform your 3-minute assessment and recognize any abnormalities.

AIRWAY AND LUNGS

The airway is divided into the upper airway and lower airway. The upper airway includes the nasopharynx (nose), oropharynx (mouth), laryngopharynx, and larynx. Its purpose is to warm, filter, and humidify inhaled air. The upper airway also helps to make sound and send air to the lower airway.

The lower airway begins with the trachea, which then divides into the right and left mainstem bronchi. The mainstem bronchi divide into the lobar bronchi, which are lined with mucus-producing ciliated epithelium, one of the lungs' major defense systems.

The lobar bronchi continue to divide until they terminate into the alveoli, the gas-exchange units of the lungs. The lungs in a typical adult contain about 300 million alveoli. The right lung is larger and has three lobes: upper, middle, and lower. The left lung is smaller and has only an upper and a lower lobe.

THORAX

The bony thorax includes the clavicles, sternum, scapula, 12 sets of ribs, and 12 thoracic vertebrae. Ribs are made of bone and cartilage and allow the chest to expand and contract during each breath.

RESPIRATORY MUSCLES

The diaphragm and the external intercostal muscles are the primary muscles

Structures of the respiratory system

The major structures of the upper and lower airway are illustrated below. The alveolus, or acinus, is shown in the inset.

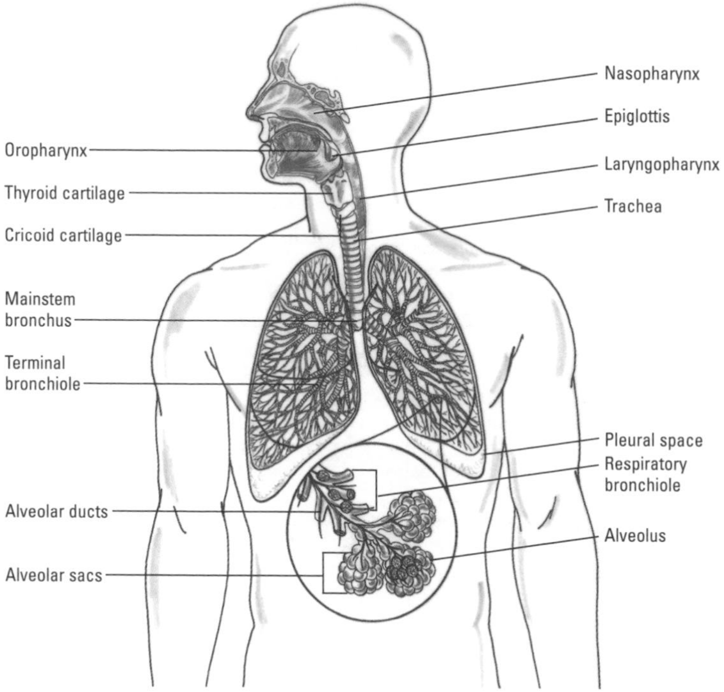

Nasopharynx

Epiglottis

Oropharynx

Laryngopharynx

Thyroid cartilage

Trachea

Cricoid cartilage

Mainstem bronchus

Terminal bronchiole

Pleural space

Respiratory bronchiole

Alveolar ducts

Alveolus

Alveolar sacs

used in breathing, contracting when the patient inhales and relaxing when the patient exhales. Other muscles that assist with breathing include the trapezius, sternocleidomastoid, and scalenes.

Essential physical assessment techniques

Any patient can develop a respiratory symptom. By using a systematic assessment, you'll be able to detect subtle or obvious respiratory changes.

The depth of your assessment will depend on several factors, including the

Respiratory system: Normal findings

Inspection
❑ Chest configuration is symmetrical side-to-side.

❑ Anteroposterior diameter is less than the transverse diameter, with a 1:2 to 5:7 ratio in an adult.

❑ Chest shape is normal, with no deformities, such as barrel chest, kyphosis, retraction, sternal protrusion, or depressed sternum. (Barrel chest may be a normal finding in infants and the elderly.)

❑ Costal angle is less than 90 degrees, with the ribs joining the spine at a 45-degree angle.

❑ Respirations are quiet and unlabored, with no use of accessory neck, shoulder, or abdominal muscles. You should also see no intercostal, substernal, or supraclavicular retractions.

❑ Chest wall expands symmetrically during respirations.

❑ Adult respiratory rate is normal, at 10 to 20 breaths/minute. Expect some variation depending on your patient's age.

❑ Respiratory rhythm is regular, with expiration taking about twice as long as inspiration. Men and children breathe diaphragmatically, whereas women breathe thoracically.

❑ Skin color matches the rest of the body's complexion.

Palpation
❑ Skin is warm and dry.

❑ No tender spots or bulges in the chest are detectable.

Percussion
❑ Resonant percussion sounds can be heard over the lungs.

Auscultation
❑ Loud, high-pitched bronchial breath sounds can be heard over the trachea.

❑ Intense, medium-pitched bronchovesicular breath sounds can be heard over the mainstem bronchi, between the scapulae, and below the clavicles.

❑ Soft, breezy, low-pitched vesicular breath sounds can be heard over most of the peripheral lung fields.

patient's primary health problem and his risk of developing respiratory complications. Keep in mind the normal assessment findings for the respiratory system. (See *Respiratory system: Normal findings*.)

A physical examination of the respiratory system involves: inspection, palpation, percussion, and auscultation. Before you begin, make sure the room is well lit and warm. The patient should be undressed from the waist up or clothed in an examination gown that allows you access to his chest.

INSPECTING THE CHEST
Examine the back of the chest first, using inspection, palpation, percussion, and auscultation. Always compare one side with the other. Then examine the front of the chest using the same sequence. The patient can lie back when you examine the front of the chest if that's more comfortable for him.

Note masses or scars that indicate trauma or surgery. Look for chest wall symmetry. Both sides of the chest should be equal at rest and expand equally as the patient inhales. The diameter of the chest, from front to back, should be about half the width of the chest.

Also, look at the angle between the ribs and the sternum at the point immediately above the xiphoid process. This angle, the costal angle, should be less than 90 degrees in an adult.

To determine the patient's respiratory rate, count for a full minute, or longer if you note abnormalities. However, don't tell him what you're doing because he might inadvertently alter his natural breathing pattern. (See *Respiration patterns,* pages 54 and 55.) Listen for audible breath sounds while inspecting.

Adults normally breathe at a rate of 10 to 20 breaths/minute. The respiratory pattern should be even, coordinated, and regular, with occasional sighs. The ratio of inspiration to expiration (I:E) is about 1:2.

Men, children, and infants usually use abdominal, or diaphragmatic, breathing. Most women, however, usually use thoracic breathing.

Watch for paradoxical, or uneven, movement of the chest wall. Paradoxical movement may appear as an abnormal collapse of part of the chest wall when the patient inhales or an abnormal expansion when the patient exhales. In either case, this uneven movement indicates a loss of normal chest wall function.

When the patient inhales, his diaphragm should descend and the intercostal muscles should contract. This dual motion causes the abdomen to push out and the lower ribs to expand laterally.

When the patient exhales, his abdomen and ribs return to their resting position. The upper chest shouldn't move much. Observe for use of accessory muscles, which may indicate a respiratory problem, particularly when the patient purses his lips when breathing. Accessory muscles may be hypertrophied, indicating frequent use.

PALPATING THE CHEST

Palpation of the chest provides important information about the respiratory system and the processes involved in breathing. Use both light and deep palpation when assessing the chest.

The chest wall should feel smooth, warm, and dry. Crepitus indicates subcutaneous air in the chest, an abnormal condition. Crepitus feels like puffed rice cereal crackling under the skin and indicates that air may be leaking from the airway or lungs.

Palpate for tactile fremitus, normal palpable vibrations caused by the transmission of air through the bronchopulmonary system. Tactile fremitus should be symmetrical. Fremitus is decreased (less intense vibrations) over areas where pleural fluid collects; at times when the patient speaks softly; and within pneumothorax, atelectasis, and emphysema. Fremitus is increased (more intense vibrations) normally over the large bronchial tubes and abnormally over areas in which alveoli are filled with fluid or exudates, as happens in pneumonia.

To check the patient for tactile fremitus, ask him to fold his arms across his chest. Lightly place your open palms on both sides of his back, without touching the back with your fingers. Ask the patient to repeat the phrase "ninety-nine" loud enough to produce palpable vibrations. Then palpate the front of the chest using the same hand positions.

Respiration patterns

Type	Description
Normal	12 to 20 breaths/minute and regular
Tachypnea	> 24 breaths/minute and shallow
Bradypnea	< 10 breaths/minute and regular
Hyperventilation	Increased rate and increased depth
Hypoventilation	Decreased rate, decreased depth, irregular pattern
Cheyne-Stokes respiration	Regular pattern characterized by alternating periods of deep, rapid breathing followed by periods of apnea
Biot's respiration	Irregular pattern characterized by varying depth and rate of respirations followed by periods of apnea

To evaluate the patient's chest wall symmetry and expansion, place your hands on the front of the chest wall with your thumbs touching each other at the second intercostal space. As the patient inhales deeply, watch your thumbs; they should separate simultaneously and equally to a distance several centimeters away from the sternum.

Repeat the measurement at the fifth intercostal space. The same measurement may be made on the back of the chest near the tenth rib.

PERCUSSING THE CHEST

You'll percuss the chest to find the boundaries of the lungs, to determine whether the lungs are filled with air, fluid, or solid material and to evaluate

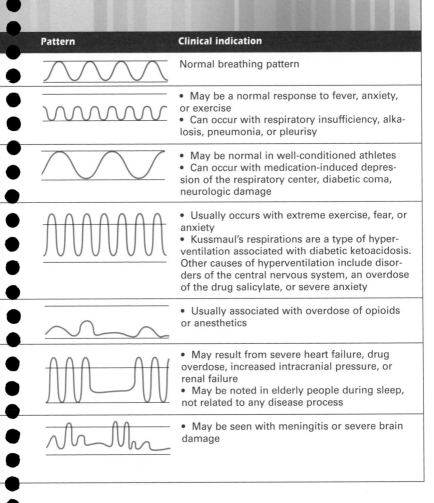

Pattern	Clinical indication
	Normal breathing pattern
	• May be a normal response to fever, anxiety, or exercise • Can occur with respiratory insufficiency, alkalosis, pneumonia, or pleurisy
	• May be normal in well-conditioned athletes • Can occur with medication-induced depression of the respiratory center, diabetic coma, neurologic damage
	• Usually occurs with extreme exercise, fear, or anxiety • Kussmaul's respirations are a type of hyperventilation associated with diabetic ketoacidosis. Other causes of hyperventilation include disorders of the central nervous system, an overdose of the drug salicylate, or severe anxiety
	• Usually associated with overdose of opioids or anesthetics
	• May result from severe heart failure, drug overdose, increased intracranial pressure, or renal failure • May be noted in elderly people during sleep, not related to any disease process
	• May be seen with meningitis or severe brain damage

the distance the diaphragm travels between the patient's inhalation and exhalation. Percussion allows you to assess structures as deep as 3″ (7.6 cm).

You'll hear resonant sounds over normal lung tissue, which you should find over most of the chest. On the front, left side of the chest, from the third or fourth intercostal space at the midclavicular line, you should hear a dull sound. Percussion is dull there because that's where the heart is. Resonance resumes at the sixth intercostal space. The sequence of sounds in the back is slightly different. (See *Percussion of lungs*, page 56.)

Percussion also allows you to assess how much the diaphragm moves during inspiration and expiration. The normal

Percussion of lungs

Percuss for tone

Starting at the apices above the scapulae, across the tops of both shoulders, percuss the intercostal spaces across and down, comparing sides. Percuss to the lateral aspects at the bases of the lungs and compare sides. Follow the sequence presented here.

Resonance (hollow) is the percussion tone elicited over normal lung tissue.

Hyperresonance (booming) is elicited in cases of trapped air such as in emphysema or pneumothorax. Dullness is present when fluid or solid tissue replaces air in the lung or occupies the pleural space. Examples include lobar pneumonia, pleural effusion, and tumor.

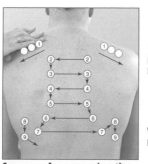

Sequence for percussing the posterior thorax

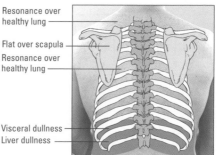

Resonance over healthy lung

Flat over scapula

Resonance over healthy lung

Visceral dullness

Liver dullness

Normal percussion tones heard from the posterior thorax

diaphragm descends 1¼" to 2" (3 to 5 cm) when the patient inhales.

AUSCULTATING THE CHEST

As air moves through the bronchi, it creates sound waves that travel to the chest wall. The sounds produced by breathing change as air moves from larger airways to smaller airways. Sounds also change if they pass through fluid, mucus, or narrowed airways.

Auscultation sites are the same as percussion sites. Listen to a full inspiration and expiration at each site, using the diaphragm of the stethoscope. Ask the patient to breathe through his mouth; nose breathing alters the pitch of breath sounds.

To auscultate for breath sounds, you'll press the stethoscope firmly against the skin. Remember that if you listen through clothing or dry chest hair, you may hear unusual and deceptive sounds.

Qualities of normal breath sounds

Breath sound	Quality	Inspiration-expiration ratio	Location
Tracheal	Harsh, high-pitched	I < E	Over trachea
Bronchial	Loud, high-pitched	I > E	Next to trachea
Bronchovesicular	Medium in loudness and pitch	I = E	Next to sternum, between scapula
Vesicular	Soft, low-pitched	I > E	Remainder of lungs

Normal breath sounds

You'll hear four types of breath sounds over normal lungs: tracheal, bronchial, bronchovesicular, and vesicular. The type of sound you hear depends on where you listen. (See *Qualities of normal breath sounds*.)

Classify each sound according to its intensity, location, pitch, duration, and characteristics. Note whether the sound occurs when the patient inhales or exhales, or both. You may also auscultate for vocal fremitus, which is a normal sound. Vocal fremitus is the sound produced by chest vibrations as the patient speaks.

Abnormal breath sounds

Adventitious (abnormal) breath sounds may be heard in the presence of respiratory symptoms. If you auscultate a normal breath sound over an area other than where you would expect to hear it, consider the sound abnormal. Other adventitious sounds are indicative of certain conditions. (See *Adventitious breath sounds,* pages 58 and 59.) Vocal fremitus may also be auscultated as an abnormal breath sound and indicates consolidation. The most common abnormal breath sounds are bronchophony, egophony, and whispered pectoriloquy. Assess the patient for abnormal vocal fremitus by auscultating over an area where you heard abnormally located bronchial breath sounds.

- *Bronchophony.* Ask the patient to say "ninety-nine" or "blue moon." Over normal lung tissue, the words sound muffled. Over consolidated areas, the words sound unusually loud.
- *Egophony.* Ask the patient to say "E." Over normal lung tissue, the sound is muffled. Over consolidated lung tissue, it sounds like the letter *a.*
- *Whispered pectoriloquy.* Ask the patient to whisper "1, 2, 3." Over normal lung tissue, the numbers are almost indistinguishable. Over consolidated lung tissue, the numbers are loud and clear.

Adventitious breath sounds

Abnormal sound	Characteristics	Source	Conditions
Discontinuous sounds			
Crackles (fine)	High-pitched, short, popping sounds heard during inspiration, and not cleared with coughing; sounds are discontinuous and can be simulated by rolling a strand of hair between your fingers and your ear.	Inhaled air suddenly opens the small deflated air passages that are coated and sticky with exudate	Crackles occuring late in inspiration are associated with restrictive diseases such as pneumonia and heart failure. Crackles occurring early in inspiration are associated with obstructive diseases such as bronchitis, asthma, or emphysema.
Crackles (coarse)	Low-pitched, bubbling, moist sounds that may persist from early inspiration to early expiration; also described as softly separating Velcro.	Inhaled air comes into contact with secretions in the large bronchi and trachea	Can indicate such conditions as pneumonia, pulmonary edema, and pulmonary fibrosis. "Velcro rales" of pulmonary fibrosis are heard louder and closer to stethoscope, usually don't change location, and are more common in clients with long-term chronic obstructive pulmonary disease.
Continuous sounds			
Pleural friction rub	Low-pitched, dry grating sound. Sound is much like crackles, only more superficial and occurs during both inspiration and expiration.	Sound is the result of rubbing of two inflamed pleural surfaces.	Pleuritis
Wheeze (sibilant)	High-pitched, musical or whistling sounds heard primarily during expiration but may also be heard on inspiration.	Air passing through constricted passages caused by swelling, secretions, or tumor.	Sibilant wheezes are often heard in cases of asthma and partial obstructive lung tissue damage.

Adventitious breath sounds (continued)

Abnormal sound	Characteristics	Source	Conditions
Continuous sounds (continued)			
Rhonchi	Low-pitched snoring or moaning sounds heard primarily during expiration but may be heard throughout the respiratory cycle. These may clear with coughing.	Air passing through secretions	Often heard in cases of bronchitis or partial obstruction and snoring before an episode of sleep apnea

Guidelines for a 3-minute assessment

A 3-minute assessment of respiratory symptoms includes making general observations, checking the patient's vital signs, and doing a brief history and performing a physical assessment based on the patient's chief sign or symptom.

MAKING GENERAL OBSERVATIONS

Observe the patient's level of consciousness (LOC), chest shape and movement, skin condition, and respiratory function.

Level of consciousness

Because the brain needs large amounts of oxygenated blood to function properly, a patient's LOC becomes a sensitive indicator of oxygenation levels. Alterations in LOC may indicate a problem in the lungs—the organs responsible for oxygenating the blood. Look for signs and symptoms of an alteration in oxygenation, such as lethargy, agitation, restlessness, increased anxiety, somnolence, confusion, or irritability.

Chest shape and movement

Examine the patient's chest for overall symmetry, shape, and appearance. In women, observe the position, location, and size of the breasts, noting deviations. Next, observe the appearance and alignment of the posterior chest, and note deviations in bony structures, such as the scapulae and the thoracic spine. Note chest deformities that may interfere with expansion. (See *Recognizing thoracic deformities,* page 60.)

Skin condition

Quickly survey the anterior and posterior chest for discoloration or breaks in skin integrity. Observe the skin of the chest area, as well as the extremities and mouth, noting cya-

Recognizing thoracic deformities

As you inspect the patient's chest, note deviations in size and shape. The illustrations here show a normal adult chest and four common chest deformities.

Normal adult chest

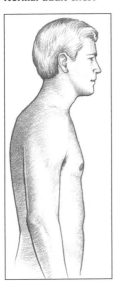

Barrel chest
Increased anteroposterior diameter

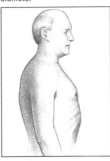

Pigeon chest
Anteriorly displaced sternum

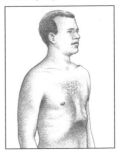

Funnel chest
Depressed lower sternum

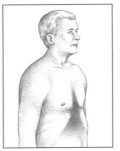

Thoracic kyphoscoliosis
Raised shoulder and scapula, thoracic convexity, and flared interspaces

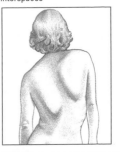

nosis, flushing, or pallor. Look for diaphoresis.

Although peripheral and central cyanosis are late signs of hypoxia, they stem from different causes. Peripheral cyanosis reflects sluggish peripheral circulation and usually results from a cardiac problem. Central cyanosis reflects excessive amounts of unsaturated hemoglobin in arterial blood, caused by inadequate oxygenation, right-to-left cardiac shunting, or a hematologic dis-

order. You'll find signs of central cyanosis in highly vascular areas, such as the lips, mouth, conjunctivae, and underside of the tongue. In dark-skinned patients, inspect the areas where cyanotic changes would be most apparent, such as the mucous membranes.

Flushing may indicate increased partial pressures of carbon dioxide in arterial blood, whereas pallor may indicate reduced oxyhemoglobin levels. Diaphoresis may indicate fever, infection, or anxiety, but it can also occur with pulmonary disorders such as pulmonary embolism. Pale, diaphoretic skin may signal early respiratory distress.

Respiratory function

Observe the patient's face for signs of pain, such as grimacing, and signs of respiratory distress, such as pursed-lip breathing or nasal flaring in pediatric patients. Does he appear short of breath or hoarse when he speaks? Do you hear signs of respiratory distress, such as crowing, wheezing, or stridor? Look at his body position. Is he leaning forward to ease breathing? Also look for accessory muscle use, and note intercostal and sternal retractions—both signs of serious breathing difficulties.

Check the rate, rhythm, and quality of the patient's respirations. If the respiratory rate is less than 10 breaths/minute, check for other changes in vital signs, a decreased LOC, and papillary constriction. If the rate is greater than 20 breaths/minute, look for signs of labored breathing. Respirations change in response to hypoxia. Initially, the body will compensate for hypoxia by increasing the respiratory rate and depth. But when the body tires, the rate and depth decrease and respiratory failure may follow. As you assess the patient's respirations, also note unusual mouth odor or sputum that may indicate an infection.

CHECKING VITAL SIGNS

If a patient complains of respiratory symptoms, continue to observe him for respiratory distress throughout your assessment. Obtain respiratory rate, temperature, heart rate, pulse oximeter, if available, and blood pressure. Assess for pain with respirations and compare all vital signs to baseline. Changes may indicate a respiratory problem or compensation for impaired gas exchange in the lungs. Patients can decompensate quickly in respiratory distress situations and vital signs may not be obtained initially.

Temperature

Fever commonly accompanies a respiratory tract infection. Gas exchange may be impaired by inflammation in the lungs. As the body fights infection, a fever may develop, causing the metabolic rate to rise and increasing oxygen demand. The combination of impaired diffusion from the infection and a fever may make it difficult to meet the body's respiratory needs.

Obtaining a temperature may be difficult if the patient is mouth breathing, tachypneic, or restless. It may be necessary to obtain a rectal or ear temperature reading.

Pulse

An elevated pulse rate may indicate hypoxia that has developed in response to sympathetic nervous system stimulation. An elevated rate may also stem from pain, fever, exertion, anxiety, or smoking.

An irregular pulse may reflect cardiac arrhythmias, especially if the patient has chronic respiratory problems and hypoxia. An irregular, thready, or weak pulse may also indicate diminished tissue and pulmonary perfusion.

Blood pressure

The patient with a respiratory problem may have normal, elevated, or depressed blood pressure. A change in blood pressure depends on the patient's previous physical condition and his ability to compensate for the existing respiratory difficulty.

If the patient has acute respiratory distress, expect his blood pressure to be normal initially, or to increase slightly to compensate for the problem. During decompensation, his blood pressure will fall.

FOCUSING ON THE CHIEF SIGN OR SYMPTOM

After you've made general observations and checked the patient's vital signs, you'll want to focus on the patient's chief respiratory sign or symptom.

Further assessment

You may need to assess another part of the body to confirm your findings or help identify the underlying cause of a problem. For instance, you may need to assess the patient's heart to determine if his sign or symptom is pulmonary or cardiac related. You may also need to assess the following:
■ neck for tracheal deviation and jugular vein distention
■ mucous membranes of the mouth and the lips for cyanosis
■ nail beds for cyanosis
■ fingers for clubbing—a sign of chronic respiratory dysfunction.

After obtaining the patient's history and performing a physical assessment, you'll begin to form a diagnostic im-

pression. (See *Respiratory system: Interpreting your findings.*)

Common signs and symptoms

A patient may seek care for any of a number of signs and symptoms related to the respiratory system. Four common ones are coughing, dyspnea, hemoptysis, and wheezing. The following assessment tips will help you assess each one quickly and accurately.

COUGHING

A cough is a sudden, noisy, forceful expulsion of air from the lungs and may be productive, nonproductive, or barking. Coughing is a necessary protective mechanism that clears airway passages. The cough reflex generally occurs when mechanical, chemical, thermal, inflammatory, or psychogenic stimuli activate cough receptors.

History

Ask the patient when the cough began and whether any body position, time of day, or specific activity affects it. Is pain associated with it? How does the cough sound—harsh, brassy, dry, croupy hacking?

If the cough is productive, find out how much sputum the patient is coughing up each day. At what time of day does he cough up the most sputum? Does his sputum production have any relationship to what or when he eats, where he is, or what he's doing? Also, ask about the color, odor, and consistency of the sputum.

Ask about cigarette, drug, and alcohol use and whether his weight or appetite has changed. Find out if he has a history of asthma, allergies, or respiratory disorders, and ask about recent illnesses, surgery, or trauma. What medications is he taking? Does he work around chemicals or respiratory irritants, such as silicone?

If a child presents with a barking cough, ask his parents if he had any previous episodes of croup syndrome. Does coughing improve upon exposure to cold air? What other signs and symptoms does the child have?

DIAGNOSTIC IMPRESSION

 Respiratory system: Interpreting your findings

Your assessment will reveal a group of findings that may lead you to suspect a particular disorder. This chart shows some common groups of findings for signs and symptoms of the respiratory system, along with their probable causes.

Sign or symptom and findings	Probable cause
Cough	
• Nonproductive cough • Pleuritic chest pain • Dyspnea • Tachypnea • Anxiety • Decreased vocal fremitus	Atelectasis
• Chronic, persistent, productive cough with small amounts of purulent (or mucopurulent), blood-streaked sputum or large amounts of frothy sputum • Dyspnea • Anorexia • Fatigue • Weight loss • Wheezing • Pain with respirations • Clubbing	Lung cancer
• Nonproductive cough • Dyspnea • Pleuritic chest pain • Decreased chest motion • Decreased to absent breath sounds • Pleural friction rub • Tachypnea • Tachycardia • Flatness on percussion • Egophony	Pleural effusion

(continued)

Respiratory system: Interpreting your findings (continued)

Sign or symptom and findings	Probable cause
Dyspnea	
• Acute shortness of breath • Tachypnea with shallow breathing • Crackles and rhonchi in both lung fields • Intercostal and suprasternal retractions • Restlessness, apprehension, motor dysfunction • Anxiety • Tachycardia • Hypoxemia despite oxygen therapy	Acute respiratory distress syndrome
• Progressive exertional dyspnea • A history of smoking • Barrel chest • Accessory muscle hypertrophy • Diminished breath sounds • Pursed-lip breathing • Prolonged expiration • Anorexia • Weight loss	Emphysema
• Tachypnea • Hemoptysis • Anxiety • Recent deep vein thrombosis • Acute dyspnea • Pleuritic chest pain • Tachycardia • Decreased breath sounds • Low-grade fever • Dullness on percussion • Cool, clammy skin	Pulmonary embolism
Hemoptysis	
• Severe cough • Sputum ranging in color from pink to dark brown • Dyspnea • Chest pain • Crackles on auscultation • Chills • Fever	Pneumonia
• Frothy, blood-tinged pink sputum • Severe dyspnea • Orthopnea • Gasping • Diffuse crackles • Cold, clammy skin • Anxiety	Pulmonary edema

Respiratory system: Interpreting your findings (continued)

Sign or symptom and findings	Probable cause
Hemoptysis (continued)	
• Night sweats • Chills • Anorexia • Chronic productive cough • Blood-streaked or blood-tinged sputum • Fine crackles after coughing • Dyspnea • Dullness to percussion • Increased tactile fremitus	Pulmonary tuberculosis
Wheezing	
• Sudden onset of wheezing • Stridor • Dry, paroxysmal cough • Gagging • Hoarseness • Decreased breath sounds • Dyspnea • Cyanosis	Aspiration of a foreign body
• Audible wheezing on expiration • Prolonged expiration • Apprehension • Intercostal and supraclavicular retractions • Rhonchi • Nasal flaring • Tachypnea • Dry cough • Hyperpnea (abnormal increases in depth and rate) • Diaphoresis • Cyanosis	Asthma
• Wheezing • Coarse crackles • Hacking cough that becomes productive • Dyspnea • Barrel chest • Clubbing • Edema • Weight gain	Chronic bronchitis

Physical assessment

Check the depth and rhythm of the patient's respirations, and note if wheezing or "crowing" noises occur with breathing. Feel the patient's skin: Is it cold, clammy, or dry? Check his nose and mouth for congestion, inflammation, drainage, or signs of infection.

Note breath odor: Halitosis can be a sign of pulmonary infection. Inspect the neck for vein distention and tracheal deviation, and palpate for masses or enlarged lymph nodes.

Observe his chest for accessory muscle use, retractions, and uneven chest expansion. Percuss for dullness, tympany, or flatness. Finally, auscultate for pleural friction rub and abnormal breath sounds, such as rhonchi, crackles, or wheezes.

Analysis

Coughing usually indicates a respiratory disorder. Your task of evaluating the cough isn't easy because the cause can range from trivial to life-threatening. It may be relatively harmless such as postnasal drip. Or the cough may stem from asthma or lung cancer.

A severe cough can disrupt daily activities and cause chest pain or acute respiratory distress. An early morning cough may indicate chronic airway inflammation, possibly from cigarette smoke. A late afternoon cough may indicate exposure to irritants. An evening cough may suggest chronic postnasal drip or sinusitis. A dry cough may signal a cardiac condition; a hacking cough, pneumonia; and a congested cough, a cold, pneumonia, or bronchitis.

Increasing amounts of mucoid sputum may suggest acute tracheobronchitis or acute asthma. If the patient has chronic productive coughs with mucoid sputum, suspect asthma or chronic bronchitis. If the sputum changes from white to yellow or green, suspect a bacterial infection.

PEDIATRIC TIP

A barking cough in children is characteristic of croup. A nonproductive cough may indicate obstruction with a foreign body, asthma, pneumonia, or acute otitis media, or it may be an early indicator of cystic fibrosis.

Because his airway is narrow, a child with a productive cough can quickly develop airway occlusion and respiratory distress from thick or excessive secretions. Causes of a productive cough in children include asthma, bronchiectasis, bronchitis, cystic fibrosis, and pertussis.

GERIATRIC TIP

Always ask elderly patients about productive or nonproductive coughing because either can indicate serious acute or chronic illness.

DYSPNEA

Usually reported as shortness of breath, dyspnea is the sensation of difficult or uncomfortable breathing. It is commonly a symptom of cardiopulmonary dysfunction. The severity varies greatly and is typically unrelated to the severity of the underlying cause. Dyspnea may arise suddenly or slowly and may subside rapidly or become chronic.

Most people normally experience dyspnea when they overexert themselves, and its severity depends on their physical condition. In a healthy person, dyspnea is quickly relieved by rest. Pathologic causes of dyspnea include pulmonary, cardiac, neuromuscular, and allergic disorders. In addition, anxiety may cause shortness of breath.

History

If your patient complains of shortness of breath, ask if it began suddenly or gradually? Is it constant or intermittent? When did the attack begin? Does it occur during activity or while at rest?

If the patient has had dyspneic attacks before, ask if they're increasing in severity. Can he identify what aggravates or alleviates these attacks? Does he have a productive or nonproductive cough or chest pain?

Ask about recent trauma, and note a history of upper respiratory tract infections, deep vein phlebitis, or other disorders.

Ask the patient if he smokes or is exposed to toxic fumes or irritants on the job.

Find out if he has orthopnea (dyspnea when in a supine position), paroxysmal nocturnal dyspnea (dyspnea during sleep), or progressive fatigue.

Physical assessment

During the physical examination, look for signs of chronic dyspnea such as accessory muscle hypertrophy (especially in the shoulders and neck). Also look for pursed-lip exhalation, clubbing, peripheral edema, barrel chest, diaphoresis, and neck vein distention. Auscultate for adventitious breath sounds, abnormal heart sounds or rhythms, egophony, bronchophony, and whispered pectoriloquy. Then palpate the abdomen for hepatomegaly.

Analysis

Dyspnea occurs when ventilation is disturbed. When ventilatory demands exceed the actual or perceived capacity of the lungs to respond, the patient becomes short of breath. Decreased lung compliance, a disturbance in the chest bellows system, an airway obstruction, or exogenous factors (such as obesity) can increase the work of breathing.

When you evaluate dyspnea, you face two tasks. First, you must determine whether the patient's dyspnea stems from cardiac or pulmonary disease. Then you must evaluate the degree of impairment the dyspnea has caused.

Your questions about the onset and severity of your patient's dyspnea should prove helpful. A sudden onset may indicate an acute problem, such as pneumothorax or pulmonary embolus. Sudden dyspnea may also result from anxiety. A gradual onset suggests a slow, progressive disorder, such as emphysema, whereas acute intermittent attacks may indicate asthma.

Precipitating factors also help pinpoint the cause. For instance, paroxysmal nocturnal dyspnea or orthopnea may stem from a chronic lung disorder or a cardiac disorder, such as left-sided heart failure. Dyspnea aggravated by activity suggests poor ventilation and perfusion or inefficient breathing mechanisms.

PEDIATRIC TIP

Normally, an infant's respirations are abdominal, gradually changing to costal by age 7. Suspect dyspnea in an infant who breathes costally, in an older child who breathes abdominally, or in any child who uses neck or shoulder muscles to help him breathe.

GERIATRIC TIP

Elderly patients with dyspnea related to chronic illness may initially not be aware of a significant change in their breathing pattern.

HEMOPTYSIS

Frightening to the patient and usually ominous, hemoptysis is the expectoration of blood or bloody sputum from the lungs or tracheobronchial tree. It's sometimes confused with bleeding from the mouth, throat, nasopharynx, or GI tract.

History

If your patient complains of hemoptysis, ask if it's mild and when it began. Has he ever coughed up blood before? About how much blood is he coughing up now? And how often?

Ask about a history of cardiac, pulmonary, or bleeding disorders. If he's receiving anticoagulant therapy, find out the drug, its dosage and schedule, and the duration of therapy. Is he taking other prescription drugs? Does he smoke?

Physical assessment

Examine the patient's nose, mouth, and pharynx to determine the source of the bleeding. Inspect the configuration of his chest, and look for abnormal movement during breathing, use of accessory muscles, and retractions. Observe respiratory rate, depth, and rhythm. Then examine the skin for lesions.

Next, palpate the patient's chest for diaphragm level and for tenderness, respiratory excursion, fremitus, and abnormal pulsations; then percuss for flatness, dullness, resonance, hyperresonance, and tympany. Finally, auscultate the lungs, noting especially the quality and intensity of breath sounds. Also auscultate for heart murmurs, bruits, and pleural friction rubs.

Obtain a sputum sample and examine it for overall quantity; for the amount of blood it contains; and for its color, odor, and consistency.

Analysis

Commonly frothy because it's mixed with air, hemoptysis is typically bright red with an alkaline pH. Expectoration of 200 ml of blood in a single episode suggests severe bleeding, whereas expectoration of 400 ml in 3 hours or more than 600 ml in 16 hours signals a life-threatening crisis.

Hemoptysis usually results from chronic bronchitis, lung cancer, or bronchiectasis. However, it may also result from inflammatory, infectious, cardiovascular, and coagulation disorders or, in rare cases, from a ruptured aortic aneurysm. In up to 15% of patients, the cause is unknown. The most common causes of massive hemoptysis are lung cancer, bronchiectasis, active tuberculosis, and cavitary pulmonary disease from necrotic infections or tuberculosis.

PEDIATRIC TIP

Hemoptysis in children may stem from Goodpasture's syndrome, cystic fibrosis or, in rare cases, idiopathic primary pulmonary hemosiderosis. Sometimes no cause can be found for pulmonary hemorrhage occurring within the first 2 weeks of life; in such cases, the prognosis is poor.

GERIATRIC TIP

If the patient is receiving anticoagulants, determine changes that need to be made in diet or medications (including over-the-counter and natural supplements) because these factors may affect clotting.

WHEEZING

Wheezes are adventitious breath sounds with a high-pitched, musical, squealing, creaking, or groaning quality. When they originate in the large airways, they can be heard by placing an unaided ear over the chest wall or at the mouth. When they originate in the smaller airways, they can be heard by placing a stethoscope over the anterior or posterior chest. Unlike crackles and rhonchi, wheezes can't be cleared by coughing.

Wheezing may be intermittent, bilateral, or unilateral, or expiratory or inspiratory.

History
Ask the patient what provokes his wheezing. Does he have asthma or allergies? Does he smoke or have a history of pulmonary, cardiac, or circulatory disorders? Does he have cancer?

Has the patient recently had surgery, illness or trauma or changes in appetite, weight, exercise tolerance, or sleep patterns?

Which drugs is he currently taking and which ones has he taken in the past? Has he been exposed to toxic fumes or respiratory irritants?

If he has a cough, ask how it sounds, when it occurs, and how often it occurs. Does he have paroxysms of coughing? Is his cough dry, sputum producing, or bloody?

Is he experiencing chest pain? If he is, determine its quality, onset, duration, intensity, and radiation. Does it increase with breathing, coughing, or certain positions?

Physical assessment
Examine the patient's nose and mouth for congestion, drainage, or signs of infection, such as halitosis. If he produces sputum, obtain a sample for examination. Check for cyanosis, pallor, clamminess, masses, tenderness, swelling, distended neck veins, and enlarged lymph nodes. Inspect his chest for abnormal configuration and asymmetrical motion, and determine if the trachea is midline. Percuss for dullness or hyperresonance, and auscultate for crackles, rhonchi, or pleural friction rubs. Note absent or hypoactive breath sounds, abnormal heart sounds, gallops, or murmurs. Also note arrhythmias, bradycardia, or tachycardia.

Analysis
Usually, prolonged wheezing occurs during expiration when bronchi are shortened and narrowed. Causes of airway narrowing include bronchospasm; mucosal thickening or edema; partial obstruction from a tumor, a foreign body, or secretions; and extrinsic pressure, as in tension pneumothorax or goiter. With airway obstruction, wheezing occurs during inspiration.

PEDIATRIC TIP
Children are especially susceptible to wheezing because their small airways allow rapid obstruction. Primary causes of wheezing include bronchospasm, mucosal edema, and accumulation of secretions. These may occur with such disorders as cystic fibrosis, acute bronchiolitis, and pulmonary hemosiderosis, or aspiration of a foreign body.

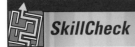
SkillCheck

1. Resonant percussion sounds are typically heard over which area?
   a. Over a solid area, as in pleural effusion
   b. Over a consolidated area, as in atelectasis
   c. Over normal lung tissue
   d. Over an area of air collection, as in a gastric air bubble or air in the intestines

Answer: c. Resonant percussion sounds (described as long, loud, low-pitched, and hollow) are typically found over normal lung tissue. You should normally find this over most of the chest.

2. Adults normally breathe at what rate?
   a. 10 to 20 breaths/minute
   b. 15 to 25 breaths/minute
   c. 22 to 30 breaths/minute
   d. 25 to 32 breaths/minute

Answer: a. The normal respiratory rate for an adult is 10 to 20 breaths/minute. The respiratory pattern should also be even, coordinated, and regular.

3. Which assessment technique allows you to assess structures as deep as 3″ (7.6 cm)?
   a. Inspection
   b. Palpation
   c. Percussion
   d. Auscultation

Answer: c. Percussion allows you to evaluate the density of deeper structures and identify the boundaries of the lung and the distance the diaphragm travels during breathing.

4. Wheezes:
   a. are high-pitched, musical, creaking breath sounds.
   b. can be cleared by coughing.
   c. can only be heard with a stethoscope.
   d. occur on inspiration only.

Answer: a. Wheezes are adventitious breath sounds with a high-pitched, musical quality that may be heard on inspiration or expiration.

5. A barking cough in children is characteristic of:
   a. asthma.
   b. bronchitis.
   c. cystic fibrosis.
   d. croup.

Answer: d. Croup causes a distinct barking cough in children.

Cardiovascular system

The cardiovascular system plays an important role in the body. As with the respiratory system, symptoms related to the cardiovascular system need immediate attention. This chapter reviews anatomy and physiology and presents the basics for a 3-minute assessment of the cardiovascular system, as well as specific history and physical assessment techniques for cardiovascular signs or symptoms.

Anatomy and physiology

The cardiovascular system delivers oxygenated blood to tissues and removes deoxygenated blood and waste products. The heart pumps blood to all organs and tissues of the body. The autonomic nervous system controls how the heart pumps. The vascular network—the arteries and veins—carries blood throughout the body, keeps the heart filled with blood, and maintains blood pressure.

Heart
The heart is a hollow, muscular organ about the size of a closed fist. It's about 5″ (12.5 cm) long and 3½″ (9 cm) in diameter at its widest point. It weighs 1 to 1¼ lb (453.5 to 567 g). The heart is located between the lungs in the mediastinum, behind and to the left of the sternum.

Anatomy of the heart
Leading in and out of the heart are the great vessels: the inferior vena cava, superior vena cava, aorta, pulmonary artery, and four pulmonary veins.

The heart has four chambers separated by the cardiac septum. The two upper chambers—the atria—have thin walls and serve as reservoirs for blood. They contract, boosting the blood into the two lower ventricles, which fill primarily by gravity. (See *Structures of the heart,* page 72.)

Blood moves to and from the heart through specific pathways. Deoxygenated venous blood returns to the right atrium through three vessels: the superior vena cava, inferior vena cava, and coronary sinus.

Blood in the right atrium empties into the right ventricle and is then ejected through the pulmonic valve into the pulmonary artery when the ventricle contracts. The blood then travels to the lungs to be oxygenated.

From the lungs, blood travels to the left atrium through the pulmonary veins. The left atrium empties the blood into the left ventricle, which then pumps the blood through the aortic valve into the aorta and throughout the body with each contraction. Because

Structures of the heart

This illustration details internal structures of the heart.

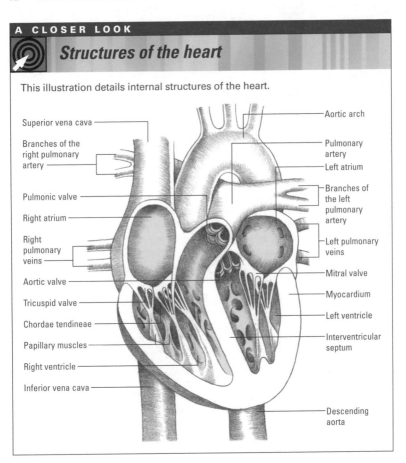

the left ventricle pumps blood against a much higher pressure than the right ventricle, its wall is three times thicker.

Valves in the heart keep blood flowing in only one direction through the heart. Healthy valves open and close passively as a result of pressure changes within the four heart chambers.

Valves between the atria and ventricles are called atrioventricular valves and include the tricuspid valve on the right side of the heart and the mitral

valve on the left. The pulmonic valve (between the right ventricle and pulmonary artery) and the aortic valve (between the left ventricle and the aorta) are called semilunar valves.

Physiology of the heart

Contractions of the heart occur in a rhythm—the cardiac cycle—and are regulated by impulses that normally begin at the sinoatrial (SA) node, the heart's pacemaker. The impulses are conducted from there throughout the heart. Impulses from the autonomic nervous system affect the SA node and alter its firing rate to meet the body's needs.

The cardiac cycle consists of systole, the period when the lower chambers of the heart contract and send blood on its outward journey, and diastole, the period when the lower chambers of the heart relax and fill with blood. During diastole, the mitral and tricuspid valves are open, and the aortic and pulmonic valves are closed. Diastole consists of ventricular filling and atrial contraction.

Systole is the period of ventricular contraction. Closure of the mitral and tricuspid valves produces the first heart sound, S_1. As the aortic and pulmonic valves snap shut, the second heart sound, S_2, is produced.

VASCULAR SYSTEM

The peripheral vascular system consists of a network of arteries, arterioles, capillaries, venules, and veins that are constantly filled, in an adult, with about $10\frac{1}{2}$ pints (5 L) of blood. The vascular system delivers oxygen, nutrients, and other substances to the body's cells and removes the waste products of cellular metabolism. (See *Arteries and veins of the body,* page 74.)

Arteries are the thick-walled, muscular vessels that carry blood away from the heart. Nearly all arteries carry oxygen-rich blood from the heart throughout the rest of the body. The only exception is the pulmonary artery, which carries oxygen-depleted blood from the right ventricle to the lungs.

The exchange of fluid, nutrients, and metabolic wastes between blood and cells occurs in the capillaries. The exchange can occur because capillaries

are thin walled and highly permeable. About 5% of the circulating blood volume at any given moment is contained within the capillary network. Capillaries are connected to arteries and veins through intermediary vessels called arterioles and venules, respectively.

Veins carry blood toward the heart. Nearly all veins carry oxygen-depleted blood, the sole exception being the pulmonary vein, which carries oxygenated blood from the lungs to the left atrium. Veins serve as a large reservoir for circulating blood. Their walls are thinner and more pliable than those of arteries to accommodate variations in blood volume.

Pulses

Arterial pulses are pressure waves of blood generated by the pumping action of the heart. All vessels in the arterial system have pulsations, but the pulsations can be felt only where an artery lies near the skin. You can palpate these peripheral pulses: temporal, carotid, brachial, radial, ulnar, femoral, popliteal, posterior tibial, and dorsalis pedis.

Physical assessment

Cardiovascular symptoms affect people of all ages and can take many forms. Using a consistent, methodical approach to your assessment will help you identify and evaluate abnormalities. (See *Cardiovascular system: Normal findings,* page 75.)

Before you begin your physical assessment, gather the necessary tools: a stethoscope with a bell and a diaphragm, an appropriate-sized blood pressure

Arteries and veins of the body

This illustration shows major arteries and veins of the body.

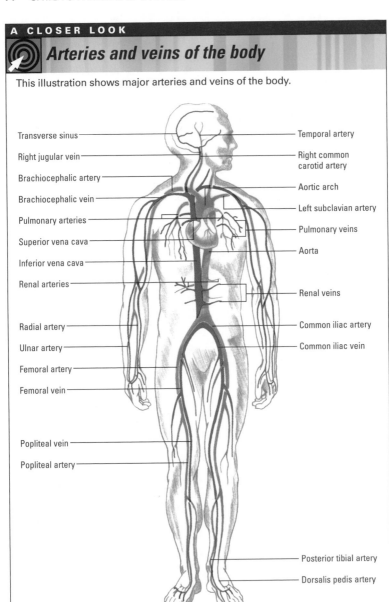

Transverse sinus

Right jugular vein

Brachiocephalic artery

Brachiocephalic vein

Pulmonary arteries

Superior vena cava

Inferior vena cava

Renal arteries

Radial artery

Ulnar artery

Femoral artery

Femoral vein

Popliteal vein

Popliteal artery

Temporal artery

Right common carotid artery

Aortic arch

Left subclavian artery

Pulmonary veins

Aorta

Renal veins

Common iliac artery

Common iliac vein

Posterior tibial artery

Dorsalis pedis artery

CHECKLIST

Cardiovascular system: Normal findings

Inspection
❑ No pulsations are visible, except at the point of maximal impulse (PMI).
❑ No lifts (heaves) or retractions are detectable in the four valve areas of the chest wall.

Palpation
❑ No vibrations or thrills are detectable.
❑ No lifts, or heaves, are detectable.
❑ No pulsations are detectable, except at the PMI and epigastric area. At the PMI, a localized (less than ½″ [1.3 cm] diameter area) tapping pulse may be felt at the start of systole. In the epigastric area, pulsation from the abdominal aorta may be palpable.

Auscultation
❑ A first heart sound (S_1):The *lub* sound is best heard with the diaphragm of the stethoscope over the mitral area when the patient is in a left lateral position. It sounds longer, lower, and louder there than a second heart sound (S_2). S_1 splitting may be audible in the tricuspid area.

❑ An S_2 sound:The *dub* sound is best heard with the diaphragm of the stethoscope in the aortic area while the patient sits and leans over. It sounds shorter, sharper, higher, and louder there than an S_1. Normal S_2 splitting may be audible in the pulmonic area on inspiration.
❑ A third heart sound (S_3) in children and slender, young adults with no cardiovascular disease is normal. It usually disappears when adults reach ages 25 to 35. In an older adult, it may signify heart failure. S_3 is heard best with the bell of the stethoscope over the mitral area with the patient in a supine position and exhaling. It sounds short, dull, soft, and low.
❑ Murmurs may be functional in children and young adults, but are abnormal in older adults. Innocent murmurs are soft, short, and vary with respirations and patient position. They occur in early systole and are best heard in pulmonic or mitral areas with the patient in a supine position.

---

cuff, a ruler, and a penlight or other flexible light source. Provide privacy and make sure the room is quiet.

Ask the patient to remove all clothing except his underwear and to put on an examination gown. Have the patient lie on his back, with the head of the examination table at a 30- to 45-degree angle. Stand on the patient's right side if you're right-handed or his left side if you're left-handed so you can auscultate more easily.

ASSESSING THE HEART
As with assessment of other body systems, you'll inspect, palpate, percuss, and auscultate in your assessment of the heart.

Inspection
First, take a moment to assess the patient's general appearance. Is he overly thin? Obese? Alert? Anxious? Note skin color, temperature, turgor, and texture. Are his fingers clubbed? (Clubbing is a sign of chronic hypoxia caused by a chronic cardiovascular or respiratory

Identifying cardiovascular landmarks

These views show where to find critical landmarks used in cardiovascular assessment.

Anterior thorax

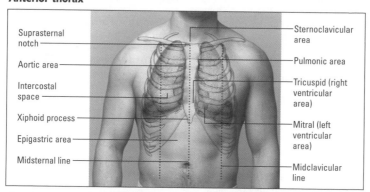

Suprasternal notch

Aortic area

Intercostal space

Xiphoid process

Epigastric area

Midsternal line

Sternoclavicular area

Pulmonic area

Tricuspid (right ventricular area)

Mitral (left ventricular area)

Midclavicular line

Lateral thorax

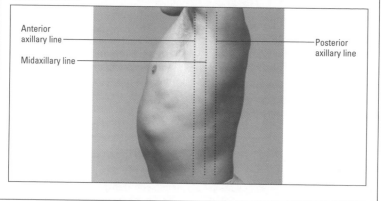

Anterior axillary line

Midaxillary line

Posterior axillary line

disorder.) If the patient is dark-skinned, inspect mucous membranes for pallor.

Next, inspect the chest. Note landmarks you can use to describe your findings, as well as structures underlying the chest wall. (See *Identifying cardiovascular landmarks.*)

Look for pulsations, symmetry of movement, retractions, or heaves. A heave is a strong outward thrust of the chest wall and occurs during systole.

Position a light source, such as a flashlight or gooseneck lamp, so that it casts a shadow on the patient's chest. Note the location of the apical impulse. This is also usually the point of maximal impulse and should be located in the fifth intercostal space medial to the left midclavicular line.

The apical impulse gives an indication of how well the left ventricle is working because it corresponds to the apex of the heart. The impulse can be seen in about 50% of adults. You'll notice it more easily in children and in patients with thin chest walls. To find the apical impulse in a woman with large breasts, displace the breasts during the examination.

Palpation

Maintain a gentle touch when you palpate so you don't obscure pulsations or similar findings. Using the ball of your hand, then your fingertips, palpate over the precordium to find the apical impulse. Note heaves or thrills, which are fine vibrations that feel like the purring of a cat.

The apical impulse may be difficult to palpate in obese and pregnant patients and in patients with thick chest walls. If it's difficult to palpate with the patient lying on his back, have him lie on his left side or sit upright. It may also be helpful to have the patient exhale completely and hold his breath for a few seconds.

Also, palpate the sternoclavicular, aortic, pulmonic, tricuspid, and epigastric areas for abnormal pulsations. Normally, you won't feel pulsations in those areas. An aortic arch pulsation in the sternoclavicular area or an abdominal aorta pulsation in the epigastric area may be a normal finding in a thin patient.

Percussion

Although percussion isn't as useful as other methods of assessment, this technique may help you locate cardiac borders. Begin percussing at the anterior axillary line, and percuss toward the sternum along the fifth intercostal space.

The sound changes from resonance to dullness over the left border of the heart, normally at the midclavicular line. The right border of the heart is usually aligned with the sternum and can't be percussed.

Percussion may be difficult in obese patients because of the fat overlying the chest or in female patients because of breast tissue. In these cases, a chest X-ray can be used to provide information about the heart border.

Auscultation for heart sounds

Cardiac auscultation requires a systematic approach and lots of practice. Begin by warming the stethoscope in your hands, and then identify the sites where you'll auscultate: over the four cardiac valves and at Erb's point, the third intercostal space at the left sternal border. Use the bell to hear low-pitched sounds and the diaphragm to hear high-pitched sounds.

Auscultate for heart sounds with the patient in three positions: lying on his back with the head of the bed raised 30 to 45 degrees, sitting up, and lying on his left side. Use a zigzag pattern over the precordium. You can start at the apex and work downward or at the base and work upward. Whichever approach you use, be consistent and keep the following tips in mind:

■ Concentrate as you listen for each sound.
■ Avoid auscultating through clothing or wound dressings because they can block sound.
■ Keep the stethoscope tubing off the patient's body and other surfaces to avoid picking up extraneous sounds.
■ Ask the patient to breathe normally. Have him hold his breath periodically to enhance sounds that may be difficult to hear.

- Use the diaphragm to listen as you go in one direction; the bell, as you come back in the other direction. Make sure you listen over the entire precordium, not just over the valves.
- Note the heart rate and rhythm.
- Always identify S_1 and S_2, and then listen for adventitious sounds, such as third and fourth heart sounds (S_3 and S_4), murmurs, and rubs.

FIRST HEART SOUND

S_1 is best heard at the apex of the heart. This sound corresponds to closure of the mitral and tricuspid valves and is generally described as sounding like *lub.* It's low pitched and dull. S_1 occurs at the beginning of ventricular systole. It may be split if the mitral valve closes just before the tricuspid.

To hear S_1, move from the base of the heart to the pulmonic area and down to the tricuspid area. Then move to the mitral area, where S_1 is the loudest.

SECOND HEART SOUND

S_2 is an extra heart sound, best heard at the base of the heart at the end of ventricular systole. This sound corresponds to closure of the pulmonic and aortic valves and is generally described as sounding like *dub.* It's a shorter, higher-pitched, louder sound than S_1.

To hear S_2, start auscultating at the aortic area, where this sound is loudest. When the pulmonic valve closes later than the aortic valve during inspiration, you'll hear a split S_2.

THIRD HEART SOUND

S_3 is an extra heart sound, best heard during diastole at the apex of the heart when the patient is lying on his left side. Often compared to the *y* sound in "Kentuck-y," S_3 is commonly heard in chil-

dren and in patients with a high cardiac output (CO). Called ventricular gallop when it occurs in adults, S_3 may be a cardinal sign of heart failure. S_3 may also be associated with such conditions as pulmonary edema, atrial septal defect, acute myocardial infarction (MI), and the last trimester of pregnancy.

FOURTH HEART SOUND

S_4 is an adventitious sound, or atrial diastolic gallop, that's heard over the tricuspid or mitral areas with the patient on his left side. Commonly described as sounding like "Ten-nes-see," S_4 occurs just before S_1, after atrial contraction. You may hear S_4 in elderly patients or patients with hypertension, aortic stenosis, or a history of an MI.

Auscultation for murmurs

A murmur is a vibrating or rumbling noise caused by turbulent blood flow through the heart valves or great vessels. Murmurs occur when structural defects in the heart's chambers or valves cause turbulent blood flow. Changes in the viscosity of blood or the speed of blood flow may also cause turbulence. Listen for murmurs over the same precordial areas used in auscultation for heart sounds.

Murmurs can occur during systole or diastole and are described by several criteria. Their pitch can be high, medium, or low. They can vary in intensity, growing louder or softer. (See *Grading murmurs.*) They can vary by location, sound pattern (blowing, harsh, or musical), radiation (to the neck or axillae), and period during which they occur in the cardiac cycle (pansystolic or midsystolic).

The best way to hear a murmur is with the patient sitting up and leaning forward. This position is best suited for hearing high-pitched sounds, such as aortic and pulmonic valve murmurs. You can also have him lie on his left side, which is best for hearing low-pitched sounds, such as mitral valve murmurs and extra heart sounds.

Auscultation for pericardial friction rub

Listening for a pericardial friction rub is also important. Have the patient sit upright, lean forward, and exhale. Listen with the diaphragm of the stethoscope over the third intercostal space on the left side of the chest. A pericardial friction rub has a scratchy, rubbing quality. If you suspect a rub but have trouble hearing one, ask the patient to hold his breath.

ASSESSING THE VASCULAR SYSTEM

Assessment of the vascular system is an important part of a full cardiovascular assessment. Examination of the patient's arms and legs can reveal arterial or venous disorders. Examine the patient's arms when you take vital signs. Check the legs later during the physical examination, when the patient is lying on his back. Remember to evaluate the patient's leg veins when he's standing.

Inspection

Start your assessment of the vascular system the same way you start an assessment of the cardiac system—by making general observations. Are the arms equal in size? Are the legs symmetrical?

Inspect the skin color. Note how body hair is distributed. Note lesions, scars, clubbing, and edema of the extremities. If the patient is confined to

---

Grading murmurs

Use the system outlined below to describe the intensity of a murmur. When recording your findings, use Roman numerals as part of a fraction, always with VI as the denominator. For instance, a grade III murmur would be recorded as "grade III/VI."

- Grade I is a barely audible murmur.
- Grade II is audible but quiet and soft.
- Grade III is moderately loud, without a thrust or thrill.
- Grade IV is loud, with a thrill.
- Grade V is very loud, with a thrust or a thrill.
- Grade VI is loud enough to be heard before the stethoscope comes into contact with the chest.

---

bed, check the sacrum for swelling. Examine the fingernails and toenails for abnormalities.

Start your inspection by observing vessels in the neck. The carotid artery should appear as a brisk, localized pulsation. The internal jugular vein has a softer, undulating pulsation. The carotid pulsation doesn't decrease when the patient is upright, when he inhales, or when you palpate the carotid. The internal jugular pulsation, on the other hand, changes in response to position, breathing, and palpation.

Check carotid artery pulsations. Are they weak or bounding? Inspect the jugular veins. Inspection of these vessels can provide information about blood volume and pressure in the right side of the heart.

To check the jugular pulse, have the patient lie on his back. Elevate the head of the bed 30 to 45 degrees and turn the patient's head slightly away from you. Normally, the highest pulsation occurs no more than $1\frac{1}{2}''$ (3.5 cm) above the sternal notch. If pulsations appear higher, it indicates elevated central venous pressure and jugular vein distention.

Palpation

The first step in palpation is to assess skin temperature, texture, and turgor. Then check capillary refill by assessing the nail beds on the fingers and toes. Refill time should be no longer than 3 seconds, or long enough to say "capillary refill."

Palpate the patient's arms and legs for temperature and edema. Edema is graded on a four-point scale. If your finger leaves a slight imprint, the edema is recorded as +1. If your finger leaves a deep imprint that only slowly returns to normal, the edema is recorded as +4.

Palpate for arterial pulses by gently pressing with the pads of your index and middle fingers. Start at the top of the patient's body at the temporal artery, and work your way down. Check the carotid, brachial, radial, femoral, popliteal, posterior tibial, and dorsalis pedis pulses.

Palpate for the pulse on each side, comparing pulse volume and symmetry. Remember not to palpate both carotid arteries at the same time; the patient could faint or become bradycardic. If you haven't put on gloves for the examination, do so when you palpate the femoral arteries.

All pulses should be regular in rhythm and equal in strength. Pulses are graded on the following scale: 4+

is bounding, 3+ is increased, 2+ is normal and easily palpable, 1+ is weak, thready, and barely palpable, and 0 is absent.

Auscultation

After you palpate, use the bell of the stethoscope to begin auscultating major vessels; then follow the palpation sequence and listen over each artery. You shouldn't hear a hum, or bruit, over the carotid arteries. A bruit sounds like buzzing or blowing and could indicate arteriosclerotic plaque formation.

Assess the upper abdomen for abnormal pulsations, which could indicate the presence of an abdominal aortic aneurysm. Finally, auscultate for the femoral and popliteal pulses, checking for a bruit or other abnormal sounds.

Guidelines for a 3-minute assessment

A 3-minute assessment of symptoms relating to the cardiovascular system includes making general observations, checking the patient's vital signs, and focusing on the patient's chief sign or symptom.

If your patient shows signs of a cardiac crisis at any point during the assessment, immediately begin emergency procedures.

MAKING GENERAL OBSERVATIONS

Your general observations will provide the first clue of a possible change in your patient's cardiac condition. Observe level of consciousness (LOC), skin condition, posture, and facial expression.

Level of consciousness
Reduced cardiac output (CO) can diminish the brain's blood flow and oxygen supply, thereby altering the patient's LOC. Be alert for signs of restlessness, agitation, and irritability. If inadequate brain oxygenation continues, the patient's LOC will deteriorate from lethargy to disorientation to confusion and, finally, to unresponsiveness.

Skin condition
Look for changes in the patient's skin color, such as pallor or cyanosis. Pallor occurs when decreased CO or increased sympathetic nervous system activity causes blood vessels to vasoconstrict, shunting blood from the skin to the heart and brain. Sympathetic vasoconstriction also causes peripheral cyanosis, seen in the nail beds, earlobes, and nose. Don't consider cyanosis alone a reliable sign of decreased oxygenation; also feel the patient's arm for warmth and dryness. If the skin feels cool or clammy, suspect peripheral vasoconstriction, possibly an early compensatory response in shock. When assessing his skin, also look for signs of edema caused by abnormal fluid accumulation in the interstitial spaces.

Posture and facial expression
Assess the patient's posture for signs of discomfort, anxiety, or labored breathing. Observe his facial expression for signs of discomfort, withdrawal, fear, or depression. Expressions of severe anxiety or impending doom should alert you to the seriousness of his situation.

Checking vital signs
Check the patient's temperature, pulse, respirations, and blood pressure and compare them with baseline vital signs. Note any deviations. Assess for pain as you check.

Temperature
Take the patient's temperature as soon as time allows. An elevated temperature may indicate cardiovascular inflammation or infection. A mild-to-moderate elevation usually occurs 2 to 5 days after an MI, as the healing infarct passes through the inflammatory stage. Acute pericarditis also may cause a similar temperature elevation. Infections, such as subacute bacterial endocarditis, cause fever spikes.

Whatever the cause, an elevated temperature always occurs with increased metabolism, which increases the cardiac workload. Therefore, you must watch feverish patients with heart disease for other signs of increased cardiac workload, such as an increased heart rate.

Pulse
Determine your patient's heart rate by assessing his radial pulse. Quickly palpating the radial pulse for 10 to 15 seconds helps you recognize gross abnormalities in rate or rhythm. As soon as possible, palpate the pulse for 1 minute to detect problems in rate or quality, especially if you suspect or know he has cardiac disease.

A weak pulse indicates either low CO or increased peripheral vascular resistance, as in arterial atherosclerotic disease. A strong, bounding pulse results from hypertension and high CO states, such as exercise, pregnancy, anemia, and thyrotoxicosis. An irregular pulse or a slow or rapid pulse may indicate an arrhythmia.

Respirations

Count your patient's respirations to determine his breathing pattern. Normally, you'll find eupnea, a regular, unlabored, and bilaterally equal breathing pattern. Tachypnea may indicate a low cardiac output. Dyspnea may indicate heart failure but isn't always evident at rest. Listen to the patient speak, and note if he must pause every few words to take a breath. A Cheyne-Stokes respiratory pattern may accompany severe heart failure, although it's more commonly associated with coma.

Blood pressure

Remember to assess your patient's blood pressure by following the techniques in chapter 1, Basic assessment review. Keep in mind that the emotional stress associated with the physical assessment may elevate a patient's blood pressure.

After measuring blood pressure, quickly calculate the pulse pressure by determining the difference between the systolic and diastolic pressures. The pulse pressure, which reflects arterial pressure during the resting phase of the cardiac cycle, normally ranges between 30 and 50 mm Hg.

The pulse pressure increases when the stroke volume (output of each ventricle at every contraction) increases, as in exercise, anxiety, or bradycardia. Pulse pressure also increases when the peripheral vascular resistance or aortic distensibility decreases, as in anemia, hyperthyroidism, fever, hypertension, aortic coarctation, or aging.

The pulse pressure decreases when a mechanical obstruction exists, such as in mitral or aortic stenosis; when the peripheral vessels constrict, as in shock; or when the stroke volume decreases, as in heart failure, hypovolemia, or tachycardia.

FOCUSING ON THE CHIEF SIGN OR SYMPTOM

After you've made general observations and checked the patient's vital signs, you'll want to focus on the patient's chief cardiovascular sign or symptom for the history and physical assessment.

Further assessment

As with the respiratory system, you may need to assess other body areas, either to gather additional information or to confirm your findings. For instance, you may want to assess the lungs because cardiac symptoms may result from a respiratory disorder.

After obtaining a history and performing the physical assessment, you'll begin to form a diagnostic impression. (See *Cardiovascular system: Interpreting your findings.*)

Cardiovascular system: Interpreting your findings

Your assessment will reveal a group of findings that may lead you to suspect a particular disorder. The chart below shows some common groups of findings for signs and symptoms of the cardiovascular system, along with their probable causes.

Sign or symptom and findings	Probable cause
Chest pain	
• A feeling of tightness or pressure in the chest described as pain or a sensation of indigestion or expansion • Pain may radiate to the neck, jaw, and arms; classically to the inner aspect of the left arm • Pain begins gradually, reaches a maximum, then slowly subsides • Pain provoked by exertion, emotional stress, or a heavy meal and relieved by rest or nitroglycerin • Pain typically lasts 2 to 10 minutes (usually no more than 20 minutes) • Dyspnea • Nausea and vomiting • Tachycardia • Dizziness • Diaphoresis	Angina
• A crushing substernal pain, unrelieved by rest or nitroglycerin • Pain that may radiate to the left arm, jaw, neck, or shoulder blades • Pain that lasts from 15 minutes to hours • Pallor • Clammy skin • Dyspnea • Diaphoresis • Feeling of impending doom	Myocardial infarction
• Sharp, severe pain aggravated by inspiration, coughing, or pressure • Shallow, splinted breaths • Dyspnea • Cough • Local tenderness and edema	Rib fracture

(continued)

Cardiovascular system: Interpreting your findings
(continued)

Sign or symptom and findings	Probable cause
Fatigue	
• Fatigue following mild activity • Pallor • Tachycardia • Dyspnea	Anemia
• Progressive fatigue • Cardiac murmur • Exertional dyspnea • Cough • Hemoptysis	Valvular heart disease
Palpitations	
• Paroxysmal palpitations • Diaphoresis • Facial flushing • Trembling • Impending sense of doom • Hyperventilation • Dizziness	Acute anxiety attack
• Paroxysmal or sustained palpitations • Dizziness • Weakness • Fatigue • Irregular, rapid, or slow pulse rate • Decreased blood pressure • Confusion • Diaphoresis	Cardiac arrhythmias
• Sustained palpitations • Fatigue • Headache • Irritability • Hunger • Cold sweats • Tremors • Anxiety	Hypoglycemia
Peripheral edema	
• Bilateral leg edema with pitting ankle edema • Weight gain despite anorexia • Nausea • Chest tightness • Hypotension • Pallor • Palpitations • Inspiratory crackles	Heart failure

Cardiovascular system: Interpreting your findings *(continued)*

Sign or symptom and findings	Probable cause
Peripheral edema *(continued)*	
• Bilateral arm edema accompanied by facial and neck edema • Edematous areas marked by dilated veins • Headache • Vertigo • Vision disturbances	Superior vena cava syndrome
• Moderate to severe, unilateral or bilateral leg edema • Darkened skin • Stasis ulcers around the ankle	Venous insufficiency

Common signs and symptoms

A patient may seek care for any of a number of signs and symptoms related to the cardiovascular system. Some common ones are chest pain, fatigue, palpitations, and peripheral edema. The following history and physical assessment tips will help you assess each one quickly and accurately.

CHEST PAIN

Chest pain can arise suddenly or gradually, and its cause may be difficult to ascertain initially. The pain can radiate to the arms, neck, jaw, or back. It can be steady or intermittent, mild or acute. And it can range in character from a sharp shooting sensation to a feeling of heaviness, fullness, or even indigestion. It can be provoked or aggravated by stress, anxiety, exertion, deep breathing, or the eating of certain foods.

Have the patient rate his pain on the 0-to-10 scale, with 0 being no pain and 10, the worst pain imaginable. Obtain a baseline pain assessment and monitor his pain for increase, change in characteristic, or relief.

Remember, cultural differences may influence how a patient expresses pain.

History

If the chest pain isn't severe, proceed with the history. Ask the patient if the pain is diffuse or in a specific area.

Sometimes a patient won't perceive the sensation he's feeling as pain, so ask whether he has any discomfort radiating to the neck, jaw, arms, or back. If he does, ask him to describe it. Is it a dull, aching, pressurelike sensation? A sharp, stabbing, knifelike pain? Does he feel it on the surface or deep inside?

Find out whether the pain is constant or intermittent. If it's intermittent, how long does it last?

Ask if movement, exertion, breathing, position changes, or the eating of certain foods worsens or helps relieve the pain. Does anything in particular seem to bring on the pain? What relieves the pain?

Review the patient's history for cardiac or pulmonary disease, chest trauma, intestinal disease, or sickle cell anemia. Find out what medications he's taking, if any, and ask about recent dosage or schedule changes.

Physical assessment

When taking the patient's vital signs, note the presence of tachypnea, fever, tachycardia, paradoxical pulse, and hypertension or hypotension. Also, look for jugular vein distention and peripheral edema. Observe the patient's breathing pattern, and inspect his chest for asymmetrical expansion. Auscultate his lungs for pleural friction rub, crackles, rhonchi, wheezing, or diminished or absent breath sounds. Next, auscultate for murmurs, clicks, gallops, or pericardial friction rub. Palpate for lifts, heaves, thrills, gallops, tactile fremitus, and abdominal mass or tenderness.

Analysis

Chest pain usually results from disorders that affect thoracic or abdominal organs, such as the heart, pleurae, lungs, esophagus, rib cage, gallbladder, pancreas, or stomach. An important indicator of several acute and life-threatening cardiopulmonary and GI disorders, chest pain can also result from musculoskeletal and hematologic disorders, anxiety, and drug therapy.

Keep in mind that cardiac-related pain may not always occur in the chest. Pain originating in the heart is transmitted through the thoracic region via the upper five thoracic spinal cord segments. Thus, it may be referred to areas served by the cervical or lower thoracic segments, such as the neck and arms. Upper thoracic segments innervate skin as well as skeletal muscles, making the origin of the pain hard to determine.

PEDIATRIC TIP
Even children old enough to talk may have difficulty describing chest pain, so watch for nonverbal clues, such as restlessness, facial grimaces, or holding of the painful area. Ask the child to point to the painful area and to where the pain goes (to find out if it's radiating). Determine the pain's severity by asking the parents if the pain interferes with the child's normal activities.

GERIATRIC TIP
Because elderly patients have a higher risk of developing life-threatening conditions—such as an MI, angina, and aortic dissection—carefully evaluate chest pain in this population. They may be stoic and not complain of pain or have decreased sense of pain.

FATIGUE

Fatigue is a feeling of excessive tiredness, lack of energy, or exhaustion accompanied by a strong desire to rest or sleep. This common symptom is distinct from weakness, which involves the muscles, but may occur with it.

History

Obtain a history to identify the patient's fatigue pattern. Ask about related symptoms and any recent viral illness or stressful changes in lifestyle.

Explore nutritional habits and appetite or weight changes.

Review the patient's medical and psychiatric history as well as family history, for chronic disorders that commonly produce fatigue.

Physical assessment

Observe the patient's general appearance for overt signs of depression or organic illness. Is he unkempt or expressionless? Does he appear tired or sickly, or have a slumped posture? If warranted, evaluate his mental status, noting especially mental clouding, attention deficits, agitation, or psychomotor retardation.

Analysis

Fatigue that worsens with activity and improves with rest generally indicates a physical disorder; the opposite pattern, a psychological disorder. Fatigue lasting longer than 4 months, constant fatigue that's unrelieved by rest, and transient exhaustion that quickly gives way to bursts of energy are other findings associated with psychological disorders.

Fatigue is a normal and important response to physical overexertion, prolonged emotional stress, and sleep deprivation. However, it can also be a nonspecific symptom of a psychological or physiologic disorder, especially viral infection and endocrine, cardiovascular, or neurologic disease.

Fatigue reflects hypermetabolic and hypometabolic states in which nutrients needed for cellular energy and growth are lacking because of overly rapid depletion, impaired replacement mechanisms, insufficient hormone production, or inadequate nutrient intake or metabolism. Cardiac causes include heart failure, an MI, and valvular heart disease.

PEDIATRIC TIP

When evaluating a child for fatigue, ask his parents if they've noticed any change in his activity level. Fatigue without an organic cause occurs normally during accelerated growth phases in preschoolage and prepubescent children. However, psychological causes of fatigue must be considered—for example, a depressed child may try to escape prob-

lems at home or school by taking refuge in sleep. In the pubescent child, consider the possibility of drug abuse, particularly hypnotics and tranquilizers.

GERIATRIC TIP

Always ask elderly patients about fatigue because this symptom may be insidious and mask more serious underlying conditions in this age-group. Temporal arthritis, which is more common in patients older than age 60, usually presents as fatigue, weight loss, jaw claudication, proximal muscle weakness, headache, vision disturbances, and associated anemia.

PALPITATIONS

Defined as a conscious awareness of one's heartbeat, *palpitations* are usually felt over the precordium or in the throat or neck. The patient may describe them as pounding, jumping, turning, fluttering, or flopping, or as missing or skipping beats. Palpitations may be regular or irregular, fast or slow, paroxysmal or sustained.

History

If the patient isn't in distress, obtain a complete cardiac history. Ask about cardiovascular or pulmonary disorders, which may produce arrhythmias. Does the patient have a history of hypertension or hypoglycemia?

Obtain a drug history. Has the patient recently started cardiac glycoside therapy? In addition, ask about caffeine, tobacco, and alcohol consumption.

Ask about associated symptoms, such as weakness, fatigue, and angina.

Physical assessment

If the patient isn't in distress, perform a complete physical assessment of the cardiovascular system. Auscultate for gallops, murmurs, and abnormal breath sounds.

To help characterize the palpitations, ask the patient to simulate their rhythm by tapping his finger on a hard surface. An irregular "skipped beat" rhythm points to premature ventricular contractions, whereas an episodic racing rhythm that ends abruptly suggests paroxysmal atrial tachycardia.

Analysis

Although frequently insignificant, palpitations are a common reason for seeking care that may result from a cardiac or metabolic disorder or from the effects of certain drugs. Nonpathologic palpitations may occur with a newly implanted prosthetic valve because the valve's clicking sound heightens the patient's awareness of his heartbeat. Transient palpitations may accompany emotional stress (such as fright, anger, and anxiety) or physical stress (such as exercise and fever). They can also accompany the use of stimulants, such as tobacco and caffeine.

PEDIATRIC TIP

Palpitations in children commonly result from fever and congenital heart defects, such as patent ductus arteriosus and septal defects. Because many children have difficulty describing this symptom, focus your attention on objective measurements, such as cardiac monitoring, physical examination, and laboratory tests.

PERIPHERAL EDEMA

The result of excess interstitial fluid in the arms or legs, peripheral edema may be unilateral or bilateral, slight or dramatic, pitting or nonpitting.

History

Begin by asking how long the patient has had the edema. Did it develop suddenly or gradually?

Does the edema decrease if the patient elevates his arms or legs? Is it worse in the mornings, or does it get progressively worse during the day?

Did the patient recently injure the affected extremities or have surgery or an illness that may have immobilized him? Does he have a history of cardiovascular disease?

Is he taking medication? Which drugs has he taken in the past?

Physical assessment

Begin the assessment by examining each extremity for pitting edema. In pitting edema, pressure forces fluid into the underlying tissues, causing an indentation that slowly fills. In nonpitting edema, pressure leaves no indentation in the skin, but the skin may feel unusually firm. Because edema may compromise arterial blood flow, palpate peripheral pulses to detect insufficiency. Observe the color of the extremity and look for unusual vein patterns. Then palpate for warmth, tenderness, and cords and gently squeeze the muscle against the bone to check for deep pain. Finally, note any skin thickening or ulceration in the edematous areas.

Analysis

Peripheral edema signals a localized fluid imbalance between the vascular and interstitial spaces. It may result from trauma, a venous disorder, or a bone or cardiac disorder.

Cardiovascular causes of arm edema are superior vena cava syndrome, which leads to slowly progressing arm edema accompanied by facial and neck edema with dilated veins marking these edematous areas, and thrombophlebitis, which may cause arm edema, pain, and warmth.

Leg edema is an early sign of right-sided heart failure. It can also signal thrombophlebitis and chronic venous insufficiency.

PEDIATRIC TIP

Uncommon in children, arm edema can result from trauma. Leg edema, also uncommon, can result from osteomyelitis, leg trauma or, rarely, heart failure.

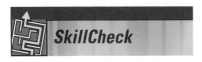

SkillCheck

1. Which statement about heart sounds is correct?
   a. S_1 and S_2 sound equally loud over the entire cardiac area.
   b. S_1 is loudest at the base; S_2, at the apex.
   c. S_1 and S_2 sound fainter at the base.
   d. S_1 is loudest at the apex; S_2, at the base.

Answer: d. Remember, S_1 is the low-pitched sound heard best at the apex; S_2, the high-pitched sound heard best at the base.

2. To best assess a patient for a pericardial friction rub, have him:
   a. lie on his right side.
   b. in a supine position and holding his breath.
   c. sitting upright, leaning forward, and exhaling.
   d. on his left side and inhaling.

Answer: c. Listen for the scratchy, rubbing sound with the patient sitting upright, leaning forward, and exhaling. Although this position brings the heart close to the chest wall, you may need to ask the patient to hold his breath if you have trouble hearing the sound.

3. How would you grade a murmur that is readily audible, but quiet and soft?
   a. Grade I/VI
   b. Grade II/VI
   c. Grade III/VI
   d. Grade IV/VI

Answer: b. Use the grading system to describe the intensity of the murmur. Grade II describes a murmur that is audible but quiet and soft.

4. Every elderly patient should be asked about:
   a. peripheral edema.
   b. fatigue.
   c. dyspnea.
   d. cough.

Answer: b. Fatigue can be insidious and mask more serious underlying conditions in patients of this age-group.

5. The nurse should suspect that the patient's pain doesn't have a cardiac origin if it radiates to:
   a. the shoulder.
   b. the jaw and neck.
   c. the arm and wrist.
   d. the abdomen.

Answer: d. Pain that originates in the heart can be transmitted through the thoracic region via the upper five thoracic spinal cord segments. Thus, it may be referred to areas served by the cervical or lower thoracic segments; however, the abdomen isn't one of these areas.

Neurologic system

The neurologic system controls body function and is related to every other body system. Consequently, patients who suffer from diseases of other body systems can develop neurologic impairments related to the disease. One example of this is a patient who has heart surgery and then suffers a stroke.

Because the neurologic system is so complex, evaluating it can seem overwhelming at first. Although tests for neurologic status are extensive, they're also basic and straightforward. In fact, your daily nursing care may routinely include some of these tests.

This chapter will help you evaluate neurologic signs or symptoms by reviewing anatomy and physiology, offering physical assessment techniques, and providing 3-minute assessment guidelines for specific signs or symptoms.

Anatomy and physiology

The neurologic system is divided into the central nervous system (CNS), the peripheral nervous system, and the autonomic nervous system. Through complex and coordinated interactions, these three parts integrate all physical, intellectual, and emotional activities.

CENTRAL NERVOUS SYSTEM
The CNS includes the brain and the spinal cord. These two structures collect and interpret voluntary and involuntary motor and sensory stimuli. (See *Structures of the central nervous system.*)

Brain
The brain consists of the cerebrum, or cerebral cortex; the brain stem, which includes the midbrain, pons, and medulla; and the cerebellum. It collects, integrates, and interprets all stimuli and initiates and monitors voluntary and involuntary motor activity. The brain is surrounded by three membrane layers called meninges and is encased by the skull.

Spinal cord
The spinal cord is the primary pathway for messages traveling between the peripheral areas of the body and the brain. The spinal cord extends from the upper border of the first cervical vertebra to the lower border of the first lumbar vertebra. It's encased by the same membrane structures as the brain and is protected by the bony vertebrae of the spine.

PERIPHERAL NERVOUS SYSTEM
The peripheral nervous system includes the peripheral and cranial nerves. Peripheral sensory nerves transmit stimuli

Structures of the central nervous system

These illustrations show a cross section of the brain and spinal cord, which together make up the central nervous system. The spinal cord joins the brain at the base of the skull and ends at the lower border of the first lumbar vertebra. Note the butterfly-shaped mass of gray matter in the spinal cord.

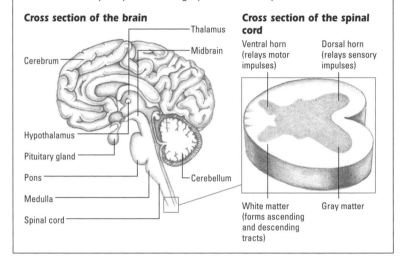

Cross section of the brain

- Thalamus
- Midbrain
- Cerebrum
- Hypothalamus
- Pituitary gland
- Pons
- Cerebellum
- Medulla
- Spinal cord

Cross section of the spinal cord

- Ventral horn (relays motor impulses)
- Dorsal horn (relays sensory impulses)
- White matter (forms ascending and descending tracts)
- Gray matter

to the spinal cord from sensory receptors in the skin, muscles, sensory organs, and viscera. The upper motor neurons of the brain and the lower motor neurons of the spinal cord carry impulses to muscles that affect movement.

The 12 pairs of cranial nerves are the primary motor and sensory pathways between the brain, head, and neck. (See *Reviewing cranial nerves,* page 92.)

AUTONOMIC NERVOUS SYSTEM

The autonomic nervous system contains motor neurons that regulate the activities of the visceral organs and affect the smooth and cardiac muscles

and the glands. It consists of two parts: the sympathetic division, which controls fight-or-flight reactions, and the parasympathetic division, which maintains baseline body functions.

Physical assessment

A complete neurologic examination is so long and detailed that you probably won't ever perform one in its entirety. However, if your initial screening examination suggests a neurologic problem, you may want to perform a more detailed assessment. (See *Neurologic system: Normal findings,* page 93.)

Reviewing cranial nerves

The cranial nerves have either sensory or motor function or both. They're assigned Roman numerals and are written: CN I, CN II, CN III, and so forth. The function of each cranial nerve is listed below.

- **CN I: Olfactory**
Smell

- **CN II: Optic**
Vision

- **CN III: Oculomotor**
Most eye movement, pupillary constriction, upper eyelid elevation

- **CN IV: Trochlear**
Down and in eye movement

- **CN V: Trigeminal**
Chewing, corneal reflex, face and scalp sensations

- **CN VI: Abducens**
Lateral eye movement

- **CN VII: Facial**
Expressions in forehead, eye, and mouth; taste

- **CN VIII: Acoustic**
Hearing and balance

- **CN IX: Glossopharyngeal**
Swallowing, salivating, and taste

- **CN X: Vagus**
Swallowing, gag reflex, talking; sensations of throat, larynx, and abdominal viscera; activities of thoracic and abdominal viscera, such as heart rate and peristalsis

- **CN XI: Accessory**
Shoulder movement and head rotation

- **CN XII: Hypoglossal**
Tongue movement

Always examine the patient's neurologic system in an orderly fashion. Begin with the highest levels of neurologic function and work down to the lowest, covering these five areas:
- mental status and speech
- cranial nerve function
- sensory function
- motor function
- reflexes.

ASSESSING MENTAL STATUS AND SPEECH

Your mental status assessment actually begins when you talk to the patient during the health history. How he responds to your questions gives clues to his orientation and memory and guides you during your physical assessment. For a quick screen of a patient's mental status, ask him the following questions:

- What's your name? (orientation to person)
- What's your mother's name? (orientation to other people)
- What year is it? (orientation to time)
- Where are you now? (orientation to place)
- How old are you? (memory)
- Where were you born? (remote memory)
- What did you have for breakfast? (recent memory)
- Who is the U.S. president? (general knowledge)
- Can you count backward from 20 to 1? (attention span and calculation skills)

The mental status examination consists of checking level of consciousness (LOC), appearance, behavior, speech, cognitive function, and constructional ability.

Neurologic system: Normal findings

Inspection

❑ Patient can shrug his shoulders, a sign of an adequately functioning cranial nerve XI (accessory nerve).

❑ Pupils are equal, round, and reactive to light, a test of cranial nerves II and III.

❑ Eyes move freely and in a coordinated manner, a sign of adequately functioning cranial nerves III, IV, and VI.

❑ The lids of both eyes close when you stroke each cornea with a wisp of cotton, a test of cranial nerve V (trigeminal nerve).

❑ Patient can identify familiar odors, a test of cranial nerve I (olfactory nerve).

❑ Patient can hear a whispered voice, a test of cranial nerve VIII (acoustic nerve).

❑ Patient can purse his lips and puff out his cheeks, a sign of an adequately functioning cranial nerve VII (facial nerve).

❑ Tongue moves easily and without tremor, a sign of a properly functioning cranial nerve XII (hypoglossal nerve).

❑ Voice is clear and strong; uvula moves upward when the patient says "ah"; gag reflex occurs when the tongue blade touches the posterior pharynx, signs of properly functioning cranial nerves IX and X.

❑ No involuntary movements are detectable.

❑ Gait is smooth.

❑ Patient is oriented to himself, other people, place, and time.

❑ Memory and attention span are intact.

❑ Deep tendon reflexes are intact.

Palpation

❑ Strength in the facial muscles is symmetrical, a sign of adequately functioning cranial nerves V and VII (trigeminal and facial nerves).

❑ Muscle tone and strength are adequate.

Level of consciousness

A change in the patient's LOC is the earliest and most sensitive indicator that his neurologic status has changed.

Clearly describe the patient's response to various stimuli using these guidelines:

■ *Alert*—follows commands and responds completely and appropriately to stimuli

■ *Lethargic*—is drowsy; has delayed responses to verbal stimuli; may drift off to sleep during examination

■ *Stuporous*—requires vigorous stimulation for a response

■ *Comatose*—doesn't respond appropriately to verbal or painful stimuli; can't follow commands or communicate verbally.

During your assessment, observe the patient's LOC. If you need to use a stronger stimulus than your voice, record what it is and how strong it needs to be to get a response from the patient. The Glasgow Coma Scale offers a more objective way to assess the patient's LOC. To use this scale, evaluate and score your patient's best eye-opening response, verbal response, and motor response. A total score of 15 indicates that he's alert; that he's oriented to time, place, and person; and that he can follow simple commands. A comatose patient will score 7 points or less. A score of 3 indicates deep coma and a poor prognosis.

EYE-OPENING RESPONSE

- Open spontaneously (Score: 4)
- Open to verbal command (Score: 3)
- Open to pain (Score: 2)
- No response (Score: 1)

VERBAL RESPONSE

- Oriented and converses (Score: 5)
- Disoriented and converses (Score: 4)
- Uses inappropriate words (Score: 3)
- Makes incomprehensible sounds (Score: 2)
- No response (Score: 1)

MOTOR RESPONSE

- Obeys verbal command (Score: 6)
- Localizes painful stimulus (Score: 5)
- Flexion, withdrawal (Score: 4)
- Flexion, abnormal, decorticate rigidity (Score: 3)
- Extension, decerebrate rigidity (Score: 2)
- No response (Score: 1)

Appearance and behavior

Also, note how the patient behaves, dresses, and grooms himself. Even subtle changes in a patient's behavior can signal the onset of an acute or chronic disorder.

Speech

Next, listen to how well the patient can express himself. Note the pace, volume, clarity, and spontaneity of speech. To assess him for dysarthria, or difficulty forming words, ask him to repeat the phrase "No ifs, ands, or buts." Assess comprehension by determining ability to follow instructions and cooperate with your examination.

Cognitive function

Assessing cognitive function involves testing the patient's memory, orientation, attention span, calculation ability, thought content, abstract thinking, judgment, insight, and emotional status. Use the mental status screening questions discussed previously to assess your patient's cognitive function.

Throughout the interview, assess the patient's emotional status. Note mood, emotional lability or stability, and the appropriateness of emotional responses. Also, assess his mood by asking how he feels about himself and his future.

Constructional ability

Constructional disorders affect the patient's ability to perform simple tasks and use various objects.

ASSESSING CRANIAL NERVE FUNCTION

The cranial nerves transmit motor or sensory messages, or both, primarily between the brain and brain stem and the head and neck. There are 12 pairs of these nerves, and all should be assessed.

- Assess cranial nerve I, the olfactory nerve, first. Make sure the patient's nostrils are patent. Have him identify the odor of at least two common substances, such as coffee, cinnamon, or cloves. Avoid stringent odors, such as ammonia or peppermint, which stimulate the trigeminal nerve.
- Next, assess cranial nerve II, the optic nerve. To test visual acuity quickly

and informally, have the patient read a newspaper, starting with large headlines and moving to small print.

Test visual fields with the confrontation technique. To do this, stand 2' (0.6 m) in front of the patient, and have him fix his gaze on you. Then bring your moving fingers forward, beginning at the periphery (6" laterally from each ear) into the patient's visual field. Ask him to tell you when he sees your moving fingers. He should see them both at the same time. Repeat the procedure with your hands at superior and inferior positions. Chart any defects you find. (See *Visual field defects*.)

Finally, examine the fundus of the optic nerve, as described in chapter 13, Eyes and ears. Blurring of the optic disk may indicate increased intracranial pressure (ICP).

■ The oculomotor nerve (cranial nerve III), the trochlear nerve (cranial nerve IV), and the abducens nerve (cranial nerve VI) all control eye movement. So assess these nerves together.

The oculomotor nerve controls most extraocular movement; it's also responsible for eyelid elevation and pupillary constriction. Abnormalities include ptosis and pupil inequality. Make sure the patient's pupils constrict when exposed to light and his eyes accommodate for seeing objects at various distances.

Also, ask the patient to follow your finger through the six cardinal positions of gaze. Forming a large H in his field of vision. Move your finger as follows: left superior, left lateral, left inferior, return to left lateral, cross over to right lateral then up to right superior, right lateral, and right inferior. Pause slightly before moving from one position to the next, to assess patient for

Visual field defects

Here are some examples of visual field defects. The black areas represent visual loss.

Left	Right
A: Blindness of right eye	
B: Bitemporal hemianopsia, or loss of half the visual field	
C: Left homonymous hemianopsia	
D: Left homonymous hemianopsia, superior quadrant	

nystagmus and the ability to hold the gaze in that particular position.

■ The trigeminal nerve (cranial nerve V) is both a sensory and motor nerve. It supplies sensation to the corneas, nasal and oral mucosa, and facial skin and supplies motor function for the jaw and all chewing muscles.

To assess the sensory component, check the patient's ability to feel light touch on his face. Ask him to close his eyes, then touch him with a wisp of cotton on his forehead, cheek, and jaw on each side. Next, test pain perception by touching the tip of a safety pin to the same three areas. Ask the patient to describe and compare both sensations.

Alternate the touches between sharp and dull to test the patient's reliability in comparing sensations. Proper assessment of the nerve requires that the patient identify sharp stimuli. To test the motor component of cranial nerve V, ask the patient to clench his teeth and then relax while you palpate the temporal and masseter muscles.

■ The facial nerve (cranial nerve VII) also has sensory and motor components. The sensory component controls taste perception on the anterior part of the tongue. You can assess taste by placing items with various tastes on the anterior portion of the patient's tongue—for example, sugar (sweet), salt, lemon juice (sour), and quinine (bitter). Simply have the patient wash away each taste with a sip of water. Taste sensation of one or more indicates functioning CN VII.

The motor component is responsible for muscles of facial expression. Assess it by observing the patient's face for symmetry at rest and while he smiles, frowns, and raises his eyebrows.

■ The acoustic nerve (cranial nerve VIII) is responsible for hearing and equilibrium. The cochlear division controls hearing; the vestibular division, balance.

To test hearing, ask the patient to cover one ear. Stand on his opposite side and whisper a few words. See whether he can repeat what you said. Test the other ear the same way.

To test the vestibular portion of this nerve, observe the patient for nystagmus and disturbed balance, and note reports of dizziness or the room spinning.

■ The glossopharyngeal nerve (cranial nerve IX) and the vagus nerve (cranial nerve X) are tested together because their innervation overlaps in the pharynx. The glossopharyngeal nerve is responsible for swallowing, salivating, and taste perception on the posterior one-third of the tongue. The vagus nerve controls swallowing and is also responsible for voice quality.

Start your assessment by listening to the patient's voice. Then check the gag reflex by touching the tip of a tongue blade against the posterior pharynx and asking him to open wide and say "ah." Watch for the symmetrical upward movement of the soft palate and uvula and for the midline position of the uvula.

■ The spinal accessory nerve (cranial nerve XI) is a motor nerve that controls the sternocleidomastoid muscles and the upper portion of the trapezius muscle. To assess this nerve, test the strength of both muscles bilaterally. First, test the sternocleidomastoid muscle by placing your palm against the patient's cheek; then ask him to turn his head against your resistance; repeat on opposite side.

Test the trapezius muscle by placing your hands on the patient's shoulders and asking him to shrug his shoulders against your resistance. During each test compare muscle strength.

■ The hypoglossal nerve (cranial nerve XII) controls tongue movement involved in swallowing and speech. The tongue should be midline, without tremors or fasciculations. Test tongue strength by asking the patient to push his tongue against his cheek as you apply resistance. Observe the tongue for symmetry. Test speech by asking him to repeat the sentence, "Round the rugged rock that ragged rascal ran."

ASSESSING SENSORY FUNCTION

Evaluation of the sensory system involves checking these five areas of sensation: pain, light touch, vibration, position, and discrimination.

Pain

To test the patient for pain, have him close his eyes; then touch all the major dermatomes, first with the sharp end of a safety pin and then with the dull end. Proceed in this order: fingers, shoulders, toes, thighs, and trunk. Ask him to identify when he feels the sharp stimulus.

If the patient has major deficits, start in the area with the least sensation, and move toward the area with the most sensation. This helps you determine the level of deficit.

Light touch

To test for the sense of light touch, follow the same routine as above, but use a wisp of cotton. Lightly touch the patient's skin. Don't swab or sweep the cotton, because you might miss an area of loss. A patient with a peripheral neuropathy might retain a sensation for light touch after he has lost pain sensation.

Vibration

To test vibratory sense, apply a tuning fork over certain bony prominences while the patient keeps his eyes closed. Apply a vibrating tuning fork to the distal interphalangeal joint of the index finger, and move proximally. Test only until the patient feels the vibration because everything above that level will be intact.

If vibratory sense is intact, you don't have to check position sense because the same pathway carries both.

Position

To assess position sense, have the patient close his eyes. Then grasp the sides of his big toe, move it up and down, and ask him what position it's in. To be tested for position sense, the patient needs intact vestibular and cerebellar function.

Perform the same test on the patient's upper extremities by grasping the sides of his index finger and moving it back and forth.

Discrimination

When testing a patient's sense of discrimination, you're assessing the ability of the cerebral cortex to interpret and integrate information. Stereognosis is the ability to discriminate the shape, size, weight, texture, and form of an object by touching and manipulating it. To test this, ask the patient to close his eyes and open his hand. Then place a common object such as a key in the hand, and ask him to identify it.

If he can't, test graphesthesia next. Have the patient keep his eyes closed and hold out his hand while you draw a large number on the palm. Ask him to identify the number. Both these tests assess the ability of the cortex to integrate sensory input.

To test point localization, have the patient close his eyes; then touch one of his limbs, and ask him where you touched him. Test two-point discrimination by touching the patient simultaneously in two contralateral areas. He should be able to identify both touches. Failure to perceive touch on one side is called extinction.

ASSESSING MOTOR FUNCTION

Assessing the motor system includes inspecting the muscles and testing muscle tone and muscle strength. Cerebellar testing is also done because the cerebellum plays a role in smooth-muscle movements, such as tics, tremors, or fasciculation.

Muscle tone

Muscle tone represents muscular resistance to passive stretching. To test arm muscle tone, move the patient's shoulder through passive range-of-motion (ROM) exercises. You should feel a slight resistance. Then let the arm drop to the patient's side. It should fall easily.

To test leg muscle tone, guide the hip through passive ROM exercises; then let the leg fall to the bed. If it falls in an externally rotated position, this is an abnormal finding.

Muscle strength

To perform a general examination of muscle strength, observe the patient's gait and motor activities. To evaluate muscle strength, ask the patient to move major muscles and muscle groups against resistance. For instance, to test shoulder girdle strength, have him extend his arms with palms up and maintain this position for 30 seconds.

If he can't maintain this position, test further by pushing down on his outstretched arms. If he does lift both arms equally, look for pronation of the hand and downward drift of the arm on the weaker side.

Cerebellar function

Cerebellar testing looks at the patient's coordination and general balance. Can he sit and stand without support? If he can, observe him as he walks across the room, turns, and walks back. Note imbalances or abnormalities.

With cerebellar dysfunction, the patient will have a wide-based, unsteady gait. Deviation to one side may indicate a cerebellar lesion on that side. Ask the patient to walk heel to toe, and observe his balance. Then perform Romberg's test: Observe the patient standing with his eyes open, feet together, and arms outstretched and then again with his eyes closed. If he falls to one side, the result of Romberg's test is positive.

Test extremity coordination by asking the patient to touch his nose and then touch your outstretched finger as you move it. Have him do this faster and faster. Movements should be accurate and smooth.

Other tests of cerebellar function assess rapid alternating movements. In these tests, the patient's movements should be accurate and smooth.

First, ask the patient to touch the thumb of his right hand to his right index finger and then to each of the remaining fingers. Observe the movements for accuracy and smoothness. Next, ask him to sit with his palms on his thighs. Tell him to turn his palms up and down, gradually increasing the speed.

Finally, have the patient lie in a supine position. Then stand at the foot of the table or bed and hold your palms near the soles of his feet. Ask him to alternately tap the sole of his right foot and the sole of the left foot against your palms. He should increase his speed as you observe his coordination. Then have him slide his right heel down the front of his left leg from knee to ankle. Repeat on the opposite side.

ASSESSING REFLEXES

Evaluating reflexes involves testing deep tendon and superficial reflexes and observing the patient for primitive reflexes.

Deep tendon reflexes

The key to testing deep tendon reflexes is to make sure the patient is relaxed and the joint is flexed appropriately. First, distract the patient by asking him to focus on a point across the room. Always test deep tendon reflexes by moving from head to toes and comparing side to side. (See *Assessing deep tendon reflexes,* page 100.)

Grade deep tendon reflexes using the following scale:

0—absent impulses
+1—diminished impulses
+2—normal impulses
+3—increased impulses, but may be normal
+4—hyperactive impulses.

Superficial reflexes

Stimulating the skin or mucous membranes is a method of testing superficial reflexes. Because these are cutaneous reflexes, the more you try to elicit them in succession, the less of a response you'll get. So observe carefully the first time you stimulate.

Using an applicator stick, tongue blade, or key, slowly stroke the lateral side of the patient's sole from the heel to the great toe. The normal response in an adult is plantar flexion of the toes. Upward movement of the great toe and fanning of the little toes—Babinski's response—is abnormal. However, this response can be elicited in some normal infants, sometimes up to age 2.

The cremasteric reflex is tested in men by using an applicator stick to stimulate the inner thigh. Normal reaction is contraction of the cremaster muscle and elevation of the testicle on the side of the stimulus.

Test the abdominal reflexes with the patient in the supine position with his arms at his sides and knees slightly flexed. Briskly stroke both sides of the abdomen above and below the umbilicus, moving from the periphery toward the midline. Movement of the umbilicus toward the stimulus is normal.

Primitive reflexes

Primitive reflexes are abnormal in adults but normal in infants, in whom the CNS is immature. As the neurologic system matures, these reflexes disappear. The primitive reflexes you'll check for are the grasp, snout, sucking, and glabella reflexes.

Assess the grasp reflex by applying gentle pressure to the patient's palm with your fingers. If he grasps your fingers between his thumb and index finger, suspect cortical or premotor cortex damage.

The snout reflex is assessed by lightly tapping on the patient's upper lip. If the lip purses, this is a positive snout reflex indicating frontal lobe damage.

Observe the patient while you're feeding him or if he has an oral airway or endotracheal tube in place. A sucking motion indicates cortical damage. This reflex is commonly seen in patients with advanced dementia.

The glabella reflex is elicited by repeatedly tapping the supraorbital ridge. The abnormal response is persistent blinking, which indicates diffuse cortical dysfunction.

Assessing deep tendon reflexes

During a neurologic examination, you assess the patient's deep tendon reflexes—that is, the biceps, triceps, brachioradialis, patellar or quadriceps, and Achilles reflexes.

Biceps reflex
Position the patient's arm so his elbow is flexed at a 45-degree angle and his arm is relaxed. Place your thumb or index finger over the biceps tendon and your remaining fingers loosely over the triceps muscle. Strike your finger with the pointed end of the reflex hammer, and watch and feel for the contraction of the biceps muscle and flexion of the forearm.

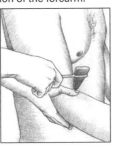

Triceps reflex
Have the patient adduct his arm and place his forearm across his chest. Strike the triceps tendon about 2" (5 cm) above the olecranon process on the extensor surface of the upper arm. Watch for contraction of the triceps muscle and extension of the forearm.

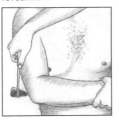

Brachioradialis reflex
Ask the patient to rest the ulnar surface of his hand on his knee with the elbow partially flexed. Strike the radius, and watch for supination of the hand and flexion of the forearm at the elbow.

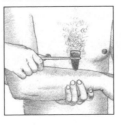

Patellar reflex
Have the patient sit with his legs dangling freely. If he can't sit up, flex his knee at a 45-degree angle, and place your nondominant hand behind it for support. Strike the patellar tendon just below the patella, and look for contraction of the quadriceps muscle in the thigh with extension of the leg.

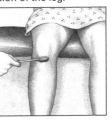

Achilles reflex
Have the patient flex his foot. Then support the plantar surface. Strike the Achilles tendon, and watch for plantar flexion of the foot at the ankle.

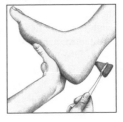

Guidelines for a 3-minute assessment

A 3-minute assessment of signs and symptoms relating to the neurologic system includes making general observations, checking the patient's vital signs, and doing a brief history and performing a physical assessment based on the patient's chief sign or symptom.

MAKING GENERAL OBSERVATIONS
Begin your assessment by checking your patient's LOC, appearance and behavior, speech, cognitive function, and constructional ability as discussed earlier in this chapter.

CHECKING VITAL SIGNS
Measure your patient's pulse, respiratory rate, and blood pressure. Findings and abnormalities may contribute to your assessment and differentiation. All are important, although changes are late indicators of changing ICP and blood flow. Also check his temperature.

FOCUSING ON THE CHIEF SIGN OR SYMPTOM
After you've made general observations and checked the patient's vital signs, you'll want to focus on the patient's chief neurologic sign or symptom for the history and physical assessment.

Further assessment

Symptoms associated with the neurologic system may affect or involve other body systems. For instance, a severely decreased LOC can affect the patient's respiratory status. Be prepared to expand your physical assessment to include other body systems.

After obtaining a history and performing the physical assessment, you'll begin to form a diagnostic impression. (See *Neurologic system: Interpreting your findings,* pages 102 and 103.)

Common signs and symptoms

A patient may seek care for any of a number of signs and symptoms related to the neurologic system. Some common ones are aphasia, decreased LOC, headache, and paralysis. The following history and physical assessment tips will help you assess each one quickly and accurately.

APHASIA
Aphasia is the impaired expression or comprehension of written or spoken language. It reflects disease or injury of the brain's language centers. Depending on its severity, it may slightly impede communication or may make it impossible.

History
If the patient doesn't display signs of increased ICP, or if aphasia has devel-

(Text continues on page 104.)

DIAGNOSTIC IMPRESSION

Neurologic system: Interpreting your findings

Your assessment will reveal a group of findings that may lead you to suspect a particular disorder. The chart below shows some common groups of findings for signs and symptoms related to the neurologic system, along with their probable causes.

Sign or symptom and findings	Probable cause
Aphasia	
• Symptoms vary with artery affected • Wernicke's, Broca's, or global aphasia • Decreased level of consciousness (LOC) • Hemiparesis or hemiplegia • Homonymous hemianopsia • Paresthesia and loss of sensation • Dysphagia	Stroke
• Any type of aphasia occurring suddenly, may be transient or permanent • Blurred or double vision • Headache • Cerebrospinal otorrhea and rhinorrhea • Cognitive impairment • Disorientation • Behavioral changes • Signs of increased ICP • Vertigo	Head trauma
• Any type of aphasia occurring suddenly and resolving within 24 hours • Transient hemiparesis • Hemianopsia • Paresthesia • Dizziness and confusion	Transient ischemic attack
Decreased LOC	
• Slowly decreasing LOC, from lethargy to coma • Apathy, behavior changes • Memory loss • Decreased attention span • Headache that's worse in the morning • Sensorimotor disturbances • Nausea and vomiting • Seizures • Focal deficits specific to tumor location • Papilledema	Brain tumor

Neurologic system: Interpreting your findings (continued)

Sign or symptom and findings	Probable cause
Headache	
• Progressive visual field loss • Acute eye pain • Blurred vision • Halo vision • Nausea and vomiting • Moderately dilated, fixed pupil	Acute angle-closure glaucoma
• Rapid, severe rise in blood pressure • Seizures • Blurred vision • Nausea and vomiting • Decreased LOC	Hypertensive crisis
• Fever, chills • Nuchal rigidity • Kernig's sign • Brudzinski's sign • Photophobia • Papilledema	Meningitis
Paralysis	
• Transient, unilateral, facial muscle paralysis • Increased tearing • Diminished or absent corneal reflex • Altered speech • Photophobia • Diminished taste • Drooling	Bell's palsy (idiopathic)
• Sporadic but progressive weakness and fatigue of skeletal muscles • May include weak eye closure, ptosis, diplopia, lack of facial mobility, and dysphagia • Neck muscle weakness • Possible respiratory distress	Myasthenia gravis
• Permanent spastic paralysis and sensory dysfunction below the level of back injury • Absent reflexes may return	Spinal cord injury

oped gradually, perform a thorough neurologic examination, starting with the patient history. You may need to obtain this history from the patient's family because of the patient's impairment.

Ask about a history of headaches, hypertension, or seizure disorders and about drug use.

Ask about the patient's ability to communicate and to perform routine activities before the aphasia began.

Physical assessment

Check for obvious signs of neurologic deficit, such as ptosis or fluid leakage from the nose and ears. Be aware that assessing the patient's LOC may be difficult because the patient's verbal responses may be unreliable. Also, recognize that dysarthria or speech apraxia may accompany aphasia, so speak slowly and distinctly, and allow the patient ample time to respond. Assess the patient's pupillary response, eye movements, and motor function, especially mouth and tongue movement, swallowing ability, and spontaneous movements and gestures. To best assess motor function, first demonstrate the motions, and then have the patient imitate them.

Analysis

Aphasia reflects damage to one or more of the brain's primary language centers, which are normally located in the left hemisphere. It can be classified as Broca's, Wernicke's, anomic, or global aphasia. Anomic aphasia eventually resolves in more than 50% of patients, but global aphasia is generally irreversible. Some causes include stroke, encephalitis, brain tumor or abscess, and head trauma.

PEDIATRIC TIP
Recognize that the term *childhood aphasia* is sometimes mistakenly applied to children who fail to develop normal language skills but who aren't considered mentally retarded or developmentally delayed. Aphasia refers solely to loss of previously developed communication skills. Brain damage associated with aphasia in children usually follows anoxia, the result of near-drowning or airway obstruction.

DECREASED LEVEL OF CONSCIOUSNESS

A decrease in LOC can range from lethargy to stupor to coma. LOC can deteriorate suddenly or gradually and can remain altered temporarily or permanently.

LOC is the most sensitive indicator of decreased neurologic function. The Glasgow Coma Scale, which measures ability to respond to verbal, sensory, and motor stimulation, can be used to quickly evaluate a patient's LOC.

History

Obtain history information from the patient if he's lucid or from his family. Did the patient complain of headache, dizziness, nausea, visual or hearing disturbances, weakness, fatigue, or any other problems before his LOC decreased?

Has his family noticed any changes in the patient's behavior, personality, memory, or temperament?

Ask about a history of neurologic disease, cancer, or recent trauma; drug and alcohol use; and the development of other signs and symptoms.

Physical assessment

Because decreased LOC can result from disorders that affect virtually every body system, tailor the remainder of your evaluation according to the patient's associated symptoms. Be sure to start by using the Glasgow Coma Scale.

Analysis

An alteration in LOC may occur gradually or as a sudden change and usually results from a neurologic disorder and commonly signals life-threatening complications of hemorrhage, trauma, or cerebral edema. However, a change in LOC can also result from a metabolic, GI, musculoskeletal, urologic, or cardiopulmonary disorder; severe nutritional deficiency; exposure to toxins; or use of certain drugs.

Consciousness is affected by the reticular activating system (RAS), an intricate network of neurons whose axons extend from the brain stem, thalamus, and hypothalamus to the cerebral cortex. A disturbance in any part of this integrated system prevents the intercommunication that makes consciousness possible. Loss of consciousness can result from a bilateral cerebral disturbance, an RAS disturbance, or both. Cerebral dysfunction characteristically produces the least dramatic decrease in a patient's LOC. In contrast, dysfunction of the RAS produces the most dramatic decrease in LOC—coma.

PEDIATRIC TIP

The primary cause of decreased LOC in children is head trauma, which commonly results from physical abuse or motor vehicle accident. Other causes include accidental poisoning, hydrocephalus, and meningitis or brain abscess following an ear or respiratory tract infection. To reduce the parents' anxiety, include them in the child's care. Offer them support and realistic explanations of their child's condition.

HEADACHE

The most common neurologic symptom, headaches, may be localized or generalized, producing mild to severe pain. About 90% of all headaches are benign and can be described as vascular, muscle contraction, or both.

History

Ask the patient to describe the headache's characteristics and location. How often does he get a headache? How long does a typical headache last?

Try to identify precipitating factors, such as certain foods and exposure to bright lights. Is the patient under stress? Has he had trouble sleeping?

Take a drug history, and ask about head trauma within the last 4 weeks.

Has the patient recently experienced nausea, vomiting, photophobia, or vision changes? Does he feel drowsy, confused, or dizzy? Has he recently developed seizures, or does he have a history of seizures?

Physical assessment

Begin the physical examination by evaluating the patient's LOC. While checking vital signs, be alert for signs of increased ICP such as a decrease in LOC. Widened pulse pressure, bradycardia, altered respiratory pattern, and increased blood pressure are late signs of increased ICP. Check pupil size and response to light, and note any neck stiffness.

Analysis

If not benign, headaches can indicate a severe neurologic disorder associated with intracranial inflammation, increased ICP, or meningeal irritation. They may also result from ocular or sinus disorders and the effects of drugs, tests, and treatments.

Other causes of headache include fever, eyestrain, dehydration, and systemic febrile illnesses. Headaches may occur with certain metabolic disturbances—such as hypoxemia, hypercapnia, hyperglycemia, and hypoglycemia—but they aren't a diagnostic or prominent symptom. Some individuals get headaches after seizures or from coughing, sneezing, heavy lifting, or stooping.

PEDIATRIC TIP

If a child is too young to describe his symptom, suspect a headache if you see him banging or holding his head. In an infant, a shrill cry or bulging fontanel may indicate increased ICP and headache. In a school-age child, ask the parents about the child's recent scholastic performance and about any problems at home that may produce a tension headache. Twice as many young boys have migraine headaches as girls. In children older than age 3, headache is the most common symptom of a brain tumor.

PARALYSIS

Bilateral or unilateral paralysis, the total loss of voluntary motor function, results from severe cortical or pyramidal tract damage. It can occur in patients with a cerebrovascular disorder, degenerative neuromuscular disease, trauma, a tumor, or a CNS infection. Acute paralysis may be an early indicator of a life-threatening disorder such as Guillain-Barré syndrome.

History

If the patient is in no immediate danger, perform a complete neurologic assessment. Start with the history, relying on family members for information if necessary.

Ask about the onset, duration, intensity, and progression of paralysis and about the events leading up to it.

Focus medical history questions on the incidence of degenerative neurologic or neuromuscular disease, recent infectious illness, sexually transmitted disease, cancer, or recent injury.

Explore related signs and symptoms, noting fever, headache, visual disturbances, dysphagia, nausea and vomiting, bowel or bladder dysfunction, muscle pain or weakness, and fatigue.

Physical assessment

Next, perform a complete neurologic examination, testing cranial nerve, motor, and sensory function and deep tendon reflexes. Assess strength in all major muscle groups, and note any muscle atrophy. Document all findings to serve as a baseline.

Analysis

Paralysis can be local or widespread, symmetrical or asymmetrical, transient or permanent, and spastic or flaccid. It's usually classified according to location and severity as paraplegia, quadriplegia, or hemiplegia. Incomplete paralysis with profound weakness, or paresis, may precede total paralysis in some patients.

PEDIATRIC TIP

Besides the obvious causes—trauma, infection, or tumors—paralysis may result from a hereditary or congenital disorder, such as Tay-Sachs disease, Werdnig-Hoffmann disease, spina bifida, or cerebral palsy.

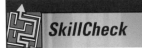

SkillCheck

1. The patient shows you he has normal tongue movement. This reflects the normal function of which cranial nerve?

    a. Cranial nerve V (trigeminal nerve)

    b. Cranial nerve VII (facial nerve)

    c. Cranial nerve X (vagus nerve)

    d. Cranial nerve XII (hypoglossal nerve)

Answer: d. Cranial nerve XII, the hypoglossal nerve, controls tongue movement.

2. What is the most common neurologic symptom?

    a. Aphasia

    b. Paresthesia

    c. Paralysis

    d. Headache

Answer: d. Headaches are the most common neurologic symptom; 90% of the time they're benign.

3. You're able to elicit a Babinski response in your 9-month-old patient. This is:

    a. a normal finding.

    b. a sign of cortical dysfunction.

    c. a sign of cerebellar dysfunction.

    d. a sign of meningeal irritation.

Answer: a. Babinski's reflex can occur normally in some infants until they reach age 2; however, in adults, it's always an abnormal response.

4. Which reflex is abnormal in an adult?

    a. Biceps reflex

    b. Brachioradialis reflex

    c. Grasp reflex

    d. Patellar reflex

Answer: c. The grasp reflex, a primitive reflex, is normal in an infant because of his immature CNS but is always abnormal in an adult.

5. What is the primary cause of decreased LOC in children?

    a. Spinal cord injury

    b. Head trauma

    c. Pneumonia

    d. Asthma

Answer: b. Head trauma, usually caused by physical abuse or a motor vehicle accident, is the primary cause of decreased LOC in the pediatric patient.

Gastrointestinal system

Gastrointestinal (GI) complaints can be especially difficult to assess and evaluate because the abdomen houses so many organs and structures, including those in the genitourinary system. An accurate 3-minute assessment is critical because GI symptoms are common, but they can also point to serious and sometimes life-threatening problems, many of which develop quickly.

This chapter spells out what you need to know to perform a 3-minute assessment of a patient with a GI symptom, from a brief anatomy and physiology review to a full physical assessment of the GI system to focusing in on specific signs or symptoms.

Anatomy and physiology

The GI system's major functions include ingestion and digestion of food and elimination of waste products. It consists of two major divisions: the GI tract and the accessory organs. (See *Structures of the GI system.*)

The GI tract is a hollow tube that begins at the mouth and ends at the anus. About 25' (7.5 m) long, the GI tract includes the pharynx, esophagus, stomach, small intestine, and large intestine.

Accessory GI organs include the liver, pancreas, gallbladder, and bile ducts. The abdominal aorta and the gastric and splenic veins also aid the GI system.

Physical assessment

A physical assessment of the GI system should include a thorough examination of the mouth and abdomen and then a thorough examination of the rectum and anus. Remember to use the following sequence when performing your assessment: inspection, auscultation, percussion, and palpation. Percussing or palpating the abdomen before auscultating can change the character of the patient's bowel sounds and lead to an inaccurate assessment. (See *GI system: Normal findings,* page 110.)

Before beginning your examination, explain the techniques you'll be using, and tell the patient that some procedures might be uncomfortable. Perform the examination in a private, quiet, warm, and well-lit room.

EXAMINING THE MOUTH

Use inspection and palpation to assess the mouth.

First, inspect the patient's mouth and jaw for asymmetry and swelling.

Structures of the GI system

This illustration shows the GI system's major anatomic structures. Knowing these structures will help you conduct an accurate physical assessment.

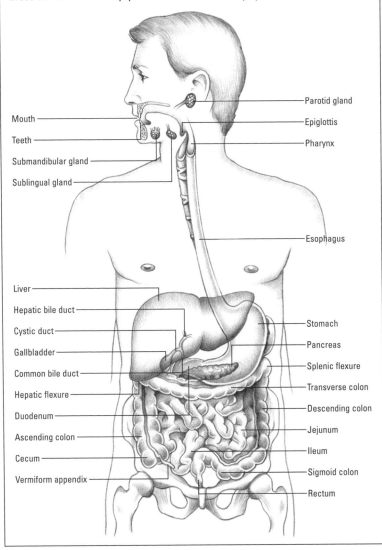

Mouth

Teeth

Submandibular gland

Sublingual gland

Liver

Hepatic bile duct

Cystic duct

Gallbladder

Common bile duct

Hepatic flexure

Duodenum

Ascending colon

Cecum

Vermiform appendix

Parotid gland

Epiglottis

Pharynx

Esophagus

Stomach

Pancreas

Splenic flexure

Transverse colon

Descending colon

Jejunum

Ileum

Sigmoid colon

Rectum

GI system: Normal findings

❏ Skin is free from vascular lesions, jaundice, surgical scars, and rashes.
❏ Faint venous patterns (except in thin patients) are apparent.
❏ Abdomen is symmetrical, with a flat, round, or scaphoid contour.
❏ Umbilicus is positioned midway between the xiphoid process and the symphysis pubis, with a flat or concave hemisphere.
❏ No variations in the color of the patient's skin are detectable.
❏ No bulges are apparent.
❏ The abdomen moves with respiration.
❏ Pink or silver-white striae from pregnancy or weight loss may be apparent.

Auscultation
❏ High-pitched, gurgling bowel sounds are heard every 5 to 15 seconds through the diaphragm of the stethoscope in all four quadrants of the abdomen.
❏ Vascular sounds are heard through the bell of the stethoscope.
❏ A venous hum is heard over the inferior vena cava.
❏ No bruits, murmurs, friction rubs, or other venous hums are apparent.

Percussion
❏ Tympany is the predominant sound over hollow organs including the stomach, intestines, bladder, abdominal aorta, and gallbladder.
❏ Dullness can be heard over solid structures, including the liver, spleen, pancreas, kidneys, uterus, and a full bladder.

Palpation
❏ No tenderness or masses are detectable.
❏ Abdominal musculature is free from tenderness and rigidity.
❏ No guarding, rebound tenderness, distention, or ascites are detectable.
❏ The liver is unpalpable, except in children. (If palpable, liver edge is regular, sharp, and nontender and felt no more than ¾" [1.9 cm] below the right costal margin.)
❏ The spleen is unpalpable.
❏ The kidneys are unpalpable, except in thin patients or those with a flaccid abdominal wall. (You'll typically feel the right kidney before you feel the left one. When palpable, the kidney is solid and firm.)

Check his bite, noting malocclusion from an overbite or underbite. Inspect the inner and outer lips, teeth, and gums with a penlight. Note bleeding, gum ulcerations, and missing, displaced, or broken teeth. Palpate the gums for tenderness and the inner lips and cheeks for lesions.

Assess the tongue, checking for coating, tremors, swelling, and ulcerations. Note unusual breath odors. Finally, examine the pharynx, looking for uvular deviation, tonsillar abnormalities, lesions, plaques, and exudate.

EXAMINING THE ABDOMEN
Use inspection, auscultation, percussion, and palpation to examine the abdomen. To ensure an accurate assessment, take these actions before the examination:
■ Ask the patient to empty his bladder.
■ If the patient is a woman, drape the genitalia and the breasts.

Abdominal quadrants

To perform a systematic GI assessment, visualize the abdominal structures by mentally dividing the abdomen into four quadrants, as shown below.

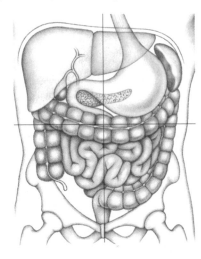

Right upper quadrant
• Right lobe of liver
• Gallbladder
• Pylorus
• Duodenum
• Head of the pancreas
• Hepatic flexure of the colon
• Portions of the ascending and transverse colon

Right lower quadrant
• Cecum and appendix
• Portion of the ascending colon

Left upper quadrant
• Left lobe of the liver
• Stomach
• Body of the pancreas
• Splenic flexure of the colon
• Portions of the transverse and descending colon

Left lower quadrant
• Sigmoid colon
• Portion of the descending colon

■ Place a small pillow under the patient's knees to help relax the abdominal muscles.
■ Keep the room warm. Chilling can cause abdominal muscles to become tense.
■ Warm your hands and the stethoscope.
■ Speak softly, and encourage the patient to perform breathing exercises or use imagery during uncomfortable procedures.
■ Assess painful areas last to help prevent the patient from becoming tense.

INSPECTING THE ABDOMEN
Begin by mentally dividing the abdomen into four quadrants and then imagining the organs in each quadrant. (See *Abdominal quadrants*.)

You can accurately pinpoint your physical findings by knowing these three terms:
■ *epigastric*—above the umbilicus and between the costal margins
■ *umbilical*—around the navel
■ *suprapubic*—above the symphysis pubis.

Observe the abdomen for symmetry, checking for bumps, bulges, or masses.

Also, note the patient's abdominal shape and contour. The abdomen should be flat to rounded in people of average weight. A protruding abdomen may be caused by obesity, pregnancy, ascites, or abdominal distention. A slender patient may have a slightly concave abdomen.

Assess the umbilicus, which should be located midline in the abdomen and inverted. Conditions such as pregnancy, ascites, or an underlying mass can cause the umbilicus to protrude. Have the patient raise his head and shoulders and inspect for protrusions.

The skin of the abdomen should be smooth and uniform in color. Note striae, or stretch marks, which can be caused by pregnancy, excessive weight gain, or ascites. New striae are pink or blue; old striae, silvery white. (In patients with darker skin, striae may be dark brown.) Also, note dilated veins. Record the length of any surgical scars on the abdomen.

Note abdominal movements and pulsations. Usually, waves of peristalsis can't be seen; if they're visible, they look like slight, wavelike motions. Visible rippling waves may indicate bowel obstruction and should be reported immediately. In thin patients, pulsation of the aorta is visible in the epigastric area.

AUSCULTATING THE ABDOMEN

Lightly place the stethoscope diaphragm in the right lower quadrant, slightly below and to the right of the umbilicus. Auscultate in a clockwise fashion in each of the four quadrants. Note the character and quality of bowel sounds in each quadrant. Make sure you listen for at least 2 minutes in each quadrant before you decide that bowel sounds are absent.

Normal bowel sounds are highpitched, gurgling noises caused by air mixing with fluid during peristalsis. The noises vary in frequency, pitch, and intensity and occur irregularly from 5 to 34 times a minute. They're loudest before mealtimes. Borborygmus is the loud, gurgling, splashing

bowel sound heard over the large intestine as gas passes through it.

Bowel sounds are classified as normal, hypoactive, or hyperactive. Hyperactive bowel sounds—loud, highpitched, tinkling sounds that occur frequently—may be caused by diarrhea, constipation, or laxative use.

Hypoactive bowel sounds are heard infrequently. They're associated with ileus, bowel obstruction, or peritonitis and indicate diminished peristalsis. Paralytic ileus, torsion of the bowel, and the use of narcotics and other medications can decrease peristalsis.

Auscultate for vascular sounds with the bell of the stethoscope. Using firm pressure, listen over the aorta and renal, iliac, and femoral arteries for bruits, venous hums, and friction rubs.

PERCUSSING THE ABDOMEN

Direct or indirect percussion is used to detect the size and location of abdominal organs and to detect air or fluid in the abdomen, stomach, or bowel.

With direct percussion, you strike your hand or finger directly against the patient's abdomen. With indirect percussion, you use the middle finger of your dominant hand or a percussion hammer to strike a finger resting on the patient's abdomen. Begin percussion in the right lower quadrant and proceed clockwise, covering all four quadrants.

If the patient has an abdominal aortic aneurysm or a transplanted abdominal organ, don't percuss the abdomen. Doing so can precipitate a rupture or organ rejection.

Percussion of the abdomen normally produces one of two sounds: tympany or dullness. Tympany is the clear, hollow, drumlike sound you hear when you percuss over hollow organs, such as an empty stomach or bowel. The sound predominates because air is normally present in the stomach and bowel. The degree of tympany depends on the amount of air and gastric dilation.

Dullness, on the other hand, is the sound you hear when you percuss over solid organs, such as the liver, kidney, or feces-filled intestines. Note where percussed sounds change from tympany to dullness.

Percussion of the liver can help you estimate its size. Hepatomegaly is commonly associated with hepatitis and other liver diseases. Liver borders may be obscured and difficult to assess. To percuss and measure the liver, follow these steps:
- Identify the upper border of liver dullness. Start in the right midclavicular line in an area of lung resonance, and percuss downward toward the liver. Use a pen to mark the spot where the sound changes to dullness.
- Start in the right midclavicular line at a level below the umbilicus, and lightly percuss upward toward the liver. Mark the spot where the sound changes from tympany to dullness.
- Use a ruler to measure the vertical span between the two marked spots, as shown. In an adult, a normal liver span ranges from $2\frac{1}{2}''$ to $4\frac{3}{4}''$ (6.5 to 12 cm).

The spleen is located at about the level of the 10th rib, in the left midaxillary line. Percussion may produce a small area of dullness, generally $7''$ (17.8 cm) or less in adults. However, the spleen usually can't be percussed because tympany from the colon masks the dullness of the spleen.

To assess a patient for splenomegaly, ask him to breathe deeply. Then per-cuss along the 9th to 11th intercostal spaces on the left, listening for a change from tympany to dullness. Measure the area of dullness. Conditions that cause splenomegaly include mononucleosis, trauma, and illnesses that destroy red blood cells, such as sickle cell anemia and some cancers.

PALPATING THE ABDOMEN

Abdominal palpation includes light and deep touch to help determine the size, shape, position, and tenderness of major abdominal organs, and to detect masses and fluid accumulation. Palpate all four quadrants, leaving painful and tender areas for last.

Light palpation helps identify muscle resistance and tenderness as well as the location of some superficial organs. To palpate, put the fingers of one hand close together, depress the skin about $\frac{1}{2}''$ (1.5 cm) with your fingertips, and make gentle, rotating movements. Avoid short, quick jabs. The abdomen should be soft and nontender.

To perform deep palpation, push the abdomen down $2''$ to $3''$ (5 to 7.5 cm). In an obese patient, put one hand on top of the other and push. Palpate the entire abdomen in a clockwise direction, checking for tenderness, pulsations, organ enlargement, and masses.

If the patient's abdomen is rigid, don't palpate it. He could have peritoneal inflammation, and palpation could cause pain or could rupture an inflamed organ.

To check the patient's liver for enlargement and tenderness, either palpate it or hook it. (See *Palpating and hooking the liver,* page 114.)

Unless the spleen is enlarged, it isn't palpable. If you do feel the spleen, stop

Palpating and hooking the liver

These illustrations show the correct hand positions for palpating and hooking the liver.

Palpating the liver
• Place the patient in the supine position. Standing at his right side, place your left hand under his back at the approximate location of the liver.
• Place your right hand slightly below the mark you made earlier at the liver's upper border. Point the fingers of your right hand toward the patient's head just under the right costal margin.
• As the patient inhales deeply, gently press in and up on the abdomen until the liver brushes under your right hand. The edge should be smooth, firm, and somewhat round. Note any tenderness.

Hooking the liver
• Hooking is an alternate way of palpating the liver. To hook the liver, stand next to the patient's right shoulder, facing his feet. Place your hands side by side, and hook your fingertips over the right costal margin, below the lower mark of dullness.
• Ask the patient to take a deep breath as you push your fingertips in and up. If the liver is palpable, you may feel its edge as it slides down in the abdomen as he breathes in.

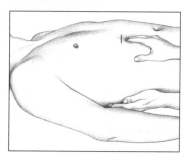 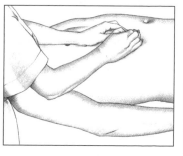

palpating immediately because compression can cause rupture.

Special assessment procedures
If you suspect peritoneal inflammation, check for rebound tenderness at the end of the examination, using the following procedure.

Choosing a site away from the painful area, position your hand at a 90-degree angle to the abdomen. Push down slowly and deeply into the abdomen, then withdraw your hand quickly. Rapid withdrawal causes the underlying structures to rebound suddenly and results in a sharp, stabbing pain on the inflamed side. If the patient has pain, don't repeat this maneuver because you may rupture an inflamed appendix.

If you suspect ascites—a large accumulation of fluid in the peritoneal cavity—use a tape measure to measure the fullest part of the abdomen. Mark this point on the patient's abdomen with indelible ink so you'll be sure to measure it consistently. This measurement is important, especially if fluid removal or paracentesis is performed.

Ascites can be caused by advanced liver disease, heart failure, pancreatitis, or cancer.

EXAMINING THE RECTUM AND ANUS

If your patient is age 40 or older, perform a rectal examination as part of your GI assessment. Make sure you explain the procedure to the patient.

First, inspect the perianal area. Put on gloves and spread the buttocks to expose the anus and surrounding tissue, checking for fissures, lesions, scars, inflammation, discharge, rectal prolapse, and external hemorrhoids. Ask the patient to strain as if he's having a bowel movement; this may reveal internal hemorrhoids, polyps, or fissures. The skin in the perianal area is normally somewhat darker than that of the surrounding area.

Next, palpate the rectum. Apply a water-soluble lubricant to your gloved index finger. Tell the patient to relax, and explain to him that he'll feel some pressure. Then insert your finger into the rectum, toward the umbilicus. To palpate as much of the rectal wall as possible, rotate your finger clockwise, then counterclockwise. The rectal walls should feel soft and smooth, without masses, fecal impaction, or tenderness.

Remove your finger from the rectum, and inspect the glove for stool, blood, and mucus. Test fecal matter adhering to the glove for occult blood using a guaiac test.

Guidelines for a 3-minute assessment

An accurate 3-minute assessment of signs or symptoms relating to the GI system depends on a well-focused history and physical assessment. Start by making general observations and checking the patient's vital signs, then focus on the patient's chief sign or symptom.

MAKING GENERAL OBSERVATIONS

Quickly survey the entire abdomen for visible deformities, and observe the patient for obvious signs of nutritional problems, such as cachexia or extreme obesity. If time and the patient's condition permit, weigh him.

Note the patient's level of consciousness (LOC). Also note facial expression, body movements, posture, and skin condition for clues to overall health status.

Level of consciousness

Assess the patient's LOC. In certain critical conditions, such as hemorrhage or perforation, decreasing LOC indicates the need for immediate intervention.

Face and body

Observe the patient's facial expression, body movements, and posture for signs of distress. Watch for signs of pain such as grimacing, writhing, clutching the abdomen, guarding, or assuming a rigid or hunched-over position. Also watch for frequent position changes, which may indicate attempts to relieve pain or discomfort.

Skin condition

Assess the patient's skin, noting color, integrity, and turgor. Pallor, diaphoresis, and cool, clammy skin may indicate internal hemorrhage. If you note these findings, quickly assess vital signs, notify the physician, and prepare to take immediate action. Dry skin and mucous membranes with poor skin turgor may indicate dehydration, requiring fluid and electrolyte replacement therapy. Jaundice, a yellowish discoloration of the skin, sclera, or mucous membranes, may point to hepatic damage or biliary obstruction.

CHECKING VITAL SIGNS

As soon as possible, obtain vital signs to establish a baseline. Then periodically monitor vital signs for changes that may signal hemodynamic alterations or an infectious process, both of which commonly affect the abdomen.

Temperature

Accurate temperature readings can help detect an early onset of fever, an important sign of infection or inflammation.

Pulse

Tachycardia may occur with shock, pain, fever, sepsis, fluid overload, or anxiety. A weak, rapid, and irregular pulse may point to hemodynamic instability, such as that caused by excessive blood loss. Diminished or absent distal pulses may signal vessel occlusion from embolization associated with prolonged bleeding.

Respirations

Altered respiratory rate and depth can result from hypoxia, pain, electrolyte imbalance, or anxiety. As with blood pressure and pulse, respiratory rate initially increases with shock. Increased respiratory rate with shallow respirations may signal fever and sepsis. Absent or shallow abdominal movement on respiration may point to peritoneal irritation.

Blood pressure

If time permits, measure blood pressure in both arms for comparison. Also, measure blood pressure with the patient lying down and sitting up, if possible.

Decreased blood pressure may signal compromised hemodynamic status, perhaps from shock caused by GI hemorrhage. Sustained, severe hypotension (systolic pressure below 70 mm Hg) results in diminished renal blood flow, which may lead to acute renal failure. Moderately increased systolic or diastolic pressure may occur with anxiety or abdominal pain. Hypertension can result from vascular damage caused by renal disease or renal artery stenosis. A blood pressure drop of greater than 30 mm Hg when the patient sits up may indicate fluid volume depletion.

FOCUSING ON THE CHIEF SIGN OR SYMPTOM

After you've made general observations and checked the patient's vital signs, you'll want to focus on the patient's chief GI sign or symptom for the history and physical assessment.

Further assessment

Because GI assessment findings can reflect problems in organs and structures outside the abdomen, you may need to assess other body regions. For example, pulmonary problems such as pneumonia and pulmonary edema can cause severe upper abdominal pain and rigidity.

After you've obtained the necessary information about the patient's chief complaint and completed your physical assessment, you'll begin to formulate a diagnostic impression. (See *GI system: Interpreting your findings,* pages 118 and 119.)

Common signs and symptoms

A patient may seek care for a number of signs and symptoms related to the GI system. The most significant ones are abdominal pain, diarrhea, hematochezia, and nausea and vomiting. The following history and physical assessment tips will help you assess each one quickly and accurately.

ABDOMINAL PAIN

Abdominal pain usually results from a GI disorder, but it can be caused by a reproductive, genitourinary, musculoskeletal, or vascular disorder; use of certain drugs; or exposure to toxins. At times, such pain may signal life-threatening complications.

History

If the patient has no life-threatening signs or symptoms, take his history. Ask if the pain is constant or intermittent and when it began. Constant, steady abdominal pain suggests organ perforation, ischemia, or inflammation or blood in the peritoneal cavity. Intermittent, cramping abdominal pain suggests the patient may have obstruction of a hollow organ.

If pain is intermittent, find out the duration of a typical episode. Also, ask the patient where the pain is located and whether it radiates to other areas.

Find out if movement, coughing, exertion, vomiting, eating, elimination, or walking worsens or relieves the pain. The patient may report abdominal pain as indigestion or gas pain, so have him describe it in detail.

Ask the patient about drug and alcohol use and history of vascular, GI, genitourinary, or reproductive disorders. If the patient is a woman, ask about the date of last menses, changes in menstrual pattern, or dyspareunia.

Ask the patient about appetite changes. Also ask about the onset and frequency of nausea or vomiting.

(Text continues on page 120.)

GI system: Interpreting your findings

Your assessment will reveal a group of findings that may lead you to suspect a particular disorder. The chart below shows some common groups of findings for signs and symptoms of the GI system, along with their probable causes.

Sign or symptom and findings	Probable cause
Abdominal pain	
• Right upper quadrant abdominal pain that may radiate between the shoulder blades • Pain may occur after eating a fatty meal • Nausea and vomiting • Chills and low-grade fever	Cholecystitis
• Localized abdominal pain, described as steady, gnawing, burning, aching, or hunger-like, high in the midepigastrium, slightly off center, usually on the right • Pain begins 2 to 4 hours after a meal • Ingestion of food or antacids brings relief • Changes in bowel habits • Heartburn or retrosternal burning	Duodenal ulcer
• Pain and tenderness in the right or left lower abdominal quadrant, may become sharp and severe on standing or stooping • Abdominal distention • Mild nausea and vomiting • Occasional menstrual irregularities • Slight fever	Ovarian cyst
• Epigastric pain • Vomiting • Abdominal rigidity • Malaise • Tachycardia	Pancreatitis
Diarrhea	
• Soft, unformed stools or watery diarrhea that may be foul-smelling or grossly bloody • Abdominal pain, cramping, and tenderness • Fever	*Clostridium difficile* infection

GI system: Interpreting your findings (continued)

Sign or symptom and findings	Probable cause
Diarrhea (continued)	
• Diarrhea occurs within several hours of ingesting milk or milk products • Abdominal pain, cramping, and bloating • Borborygmi • Flatus	Lactose intolerance
• Recurrent bloody diarrhea that may contain pus or mucus • Hyperactive bowel sounds • Cramping lower abdominal pain • Occasional nausea and vomiting • Weakness	Ulcerative colitis
Hematochezia	
• Moderate to severe rectal bleeding • Epistaxis • Purpura	Coagulation disorders
• Bright-red rectal bleeding with or without pain • Diarrhea or ribbon-shaped stools • Stools may be grossly bloody • Weakness and fatigue • Abdominal aching and dull cramps	Colon cancer
• Chronic bleeding with defecation • Painful defecation	Hemorrhoids
Nausea and vomiting	
• Nausea and vomiting follow or accompany abdominal pain • Pain progresses rapidly to severe, stabbing pain in the right lower quadrant (McBurney's sign) • Abdominal rigidity and tenderness • Constipation or diarrhea • Tachycardia	Appendicitis
• Nausea and vomiting of undigested food • Diarrhea • Abdominal cramping or pain • Hyperactive bowel sounds • Fever • Malaise	Gastroenteritis

Find out about any changes in bowel habits, such as constipation, diarrhea, and changes in stool consistency. When was the last bowel movement? Ask about urinary frequency, urgency, or pain. Is the urine cloudy or pink?

Physical assessment

Assess skin turgor and mucous membranes. Inspect his abdomen for distention or visible peristaltic waves and, if indicated, measure abdominal girth.

Auscultate for bowel sounds, and characterize their motility. Percuss all quadrants, carefully noting the percussion sounds. Palpate the entire abdomen for masses, rigidity, and tenderness. Check specifically for costovertebral angle tenderness, abdominal tenderness with guarding, and rebound tenderness.

Analysis

Abdominal pain arises from the abdominopelvic viscera, the parietal peritoneum, or from the capsules of the liver, kidney, or spleen, and may be acute or chronic, diffuse, or localized. Visceral pain develops slowly into a deep, dull, aching pain that's poorly localized in the epigastric, periumbilical, or hypogastric regions. In contrast, somatic—parietal or peritoneal—pain produces a sharp, more intense, and well-localized discomfort that rapidly follows the insult. Movement or coughing aggravates this pain.

Pain may also be referred to the abdomen from another site with the same or similar nerve supply. This sharp, well-localized, referred pain is felt in skin or deeper tissues and may coexist with skin hyperesthesia and muscle hyperalgesia.

Mechanisms that produce abdominal pain include stretching or tension of the gut wall, traction on the peritoneum or mesentery, vigorous intestinal contraction, inflammation, ischemia, and sensory nerve irritation.

PEDIATRIC TIP
Because many children have difficulty describing abdominal pain, you should pay close attention to nonverbal cues, such as wincing, lethargy, or unusual positioning (such as a side-lying position with knees flexed to the abdomen). Observing the child while he coughs, walks, or climbs may offer some diagnostic clues. Also, remember that a parent's description of the child's complaints is a subjective interpretation of what the parent believes is wrong.

In children, abdominal pain can signal a disorder with greater severity or different associated signs than in adults. Appendicitis, for example, has a higher rupture rate and mortality in children, and vomiting may be the only other sign. Acute pyelonephritis may cause abdominal pain, vomiting, and diarrhea, but not the classic urologic signs found in adults. Peptic ulcer, which is becoming increasingly common in teenagers, causes nocturnal pain and colic that, unlike peptic ulcer in adults, may not be relieved by food.

Abdominal pain in children can also result from lactose intolerance, allergic-tension-fatigue syndrome, volvulus, Meckel's diverticulum, intussusception, mesenteric adenitis, diabetes mellitus, juvenile rheumatoid arthritis, or an uncommon disorder such as heavy metal poisoning. Remember, that a child's complaint of abdominal pain may also reflect an emotional need, such as a wish to avoid school or to gain adult attention.

GERIATRIC TIP

Advanced age may decrease the symptoms of acute abdominal disease. Pain may be less severe (or the patient may be stoic about pain), fever less pronounced, and signs of peritoneal inflammation diminished or absent.

DIARRHEA

Usually a chief sign of an intestinal disorder, diarrhea is an increase in the volume, frequency, and liquidity of stools compared with the patient's normal bowel habits. It varies in severity and may be acute or chronic.

History

Begin by exploring signs and symptoms associated with diarrhea. Does the patient have abdominal pain and cramps? Difficulty breathing? Is he weak or fatigued?

Find out his drug history. Has he had recent GI surgery or radiation therapy?

Ask the patient to briefly describe his diet. Does he have any known food allergies? Last, find out if he's under unusual stress.

Physical assessment

If the patient isn't in shock, proceed with a brief physical examination. Evaluate hydration, check skin turgor, and take blood pressure with the patient lying, sitting, and standing. Inspect the abdomen for distention, and palpate for tenderness. Auscultate bowel sounds. Take the patient's temperature, and note any chills. Also, look for a rash. Conduct a rectal examination and a pelvic examination if indicated.

Analysis

Acute diarrhea may result from acute infection, stress, fecal impaction, or use of certain drugs. Chronic diarrhea may result from chronic infection, obstructive and inflammatory bowel disease, malabsorption syndrome, an endocrine disorder, or GI surgery. Periodic diarrhea may result from food intolerance or from ingestion of spicy or high-fiber foods or caffeine.

One or more pathophysiologic mechanisms may contribute to diarrhea. The fluid and electrolyte imbalances it produces may precipitate life-threatening arrhythmias or hypovolemic shock.

PEDIATRIC TIP

Diarrhea in children commonly results from infection, although chronic diarrhea may result from malabsorption syndrome, an anatomic defect, or allergies. Because dehydration and electrolyte imbalance occur rapidly in children, diarrhea can be life-threatening. Diligently monitor all episodes of diarrhea, and replace fluids immediately.

GERIATRIC TIP

In the elderly patient with new-onset segmental colitis, always consider ischemia before labeling the patient as having Crohn's disease.

HEMATOCHEZIA

Hematochezia, or the passage of bloody stools, usually indicates—and may be the first sign of—GI bleeding below the ligament of Treitz. Usually preceded by hematemesis, this sign may also accompany rapid hemorrhage of 1 L or more from the upper GI tract.

Hematochezia ranges from formed, blood-streaked stools to liquid, bloody stools that may be bright-red, dark mahogany, or maroon in color. This sign usually develops abruptly and is heralded by abdominal pain.

History

If the hematochezia isn't immediately life-threatening, ask the patient to fully describe the amount, color, and consistency of bloody stools. (If possible, also inspect and characterize the stools yourself.)

How long have the stools been bloody? Do they always look the same or does the amount of blood seem to vary? Ask about associated symptoms.

Explore the patient's medical history, focusing on GI and coagulation disorders.

Ask about use of GI irritants, such as alcohol, aspirin, and other nonsteroidal anti-inflammatory drugs.

Physical assessment

Begin the physical examination by checking for orthostatic hypotension, an early sign of shock. Take the patient's blood pressure and pulse while he's lying down, sitting, and standing. If systolic pressure decreases by 10 mm Hg or more or if pulse rate increases by 10 beats/minute or more when he changes position, suspect volume depletion and impending shock.

Examine the skin for petechiae or spider angiomas. Palpate the abdomen for tenderness, pain, or masses. Also, note lymphadenopathy. Finally, perform a digital rectal examination to rule out any rectal masses.

Analysis

Although hematochezia is commonly associated with GI disorders, it may also result from a coagulation disorder, exposure to toxins, or a diagnostic test. Always a significant sign, hemato-

chezia may precipitate life-threatening hypovolemia.

PEDIATRIC TIP

Hematochezia is much less common in children than in adults. It may result from a structural disorder, such as intussusception or Meckel's diverticulum, or from inflammatory disorders, such as peptic ulcer disease and ulcerative colitis. In children, ulcerative colitis typically produces chronic, rather than acute, signs and symptoms and may also cause slow growth and maturation related to malnutrition. Suspect sexual abuse in all cases of rectal bleeding in children.

GERIATRIC TIP

Because elderly patients are at increased risk for colon cancer, hematochezia should be evaluated with colonoscopy after perirectal lesions have been ruled out as the cause of bleeding.

NAUSEA AND VOMITING

Nausea is a sensation of profound revulsion to food or of impending vomiting. Typically accompanied by autonomic signs—such as hypersalivation, diaphoresis, tachycardia, pallor, and tachypnea—it's closely associated with vomiting.

Vomiting is the forceful expulsion of gastric contents through the mouth. Characteristically preceded by nausea, vomiting results from a coordinated sequence of abdominal muscle contractions and reverse esophageal peristalsis.

History

Begin by obtaining a complete medical history, focusing on GI, endocrine, and metabolic disorders, recent infections, and cancer and its treatment.

Ask your patient to describe the onset, duration, and intensity of nausea and vomiting. What started it? What makes it subside? Does he always experience both together?

Explore related complaints, particularly abdominal pain, anorexia and weight loss, changes in bowel habits or stools, excessive belching or flatus, and bloating or fullness.

If possible, collect, measure, and inspect the character of the vomitus, or have the patient describe it to you.

If the patient is a woman, ask if she is or could be pregnant.

Physical assessment
Inspect the skin for jaundice, bruises, and spider hemangiomas, and assess skin turgor. Inspect the abdomen for distention, and auscultate for bowel sounds and bruits. Palpate for rigidity and tenderness, and test for rebound tenderness. Next, palpate and percuss the liver for enlargement. Assess other body systems as appropriate.

Analysis
Nausea and vomiting, common indications of a GI disorder, also occur with fluid and electrolyte imbalance; infection; metabolic, endocrine, labyrinthine, and cardiac disorders; use of certain drugs; surgery; and radiation.

Often present during the first trimester of pregnancy, nausea and vomiting may also arise from severe pain, anxiety, alcohol intoxication, overeating, or ingestion of distasteful food or liquids.

PEDIATRIC TIP
Nausea, commonly described as stomachache, is one of the most common childhood complaints. It can result from overeating or from any of several diverse disorders, ranging from an acute infection to a conversion reaction caused by fear.

In a neonate, pyloric obstruction may cause projectile vomiting, whereas Hirschsprung's disease may cause fecal vomiting. Intussusception may lead to vomiting of bile and fecal matter in an infant or toddler. Because an infant may aspirate vomitus as a result of immature cough and gag reflexes, position him on his side or abdomen, and clear any vomitus immediately.

GERIATRIC TIP
Elderly patients have increased dental caries; tooth loss; decreased salivary gland function, which causes mouth dryness; decreased gastric acid output and motility; and decreased sense of taste and smell. And, all of these can contribute to nonpathologic nausea. However, intestinal ischemia, which is common in this age-group, should always be ruled out as a potential cause for nausea and vomiting.

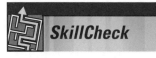

SkillCheck

1. Hyperactive bowel sounds can result from all of the following except:
   a. diarrhea.
   b. laxative use.
   c. constipation.
   d. ileus.
Answer: d. Hypoactive, not hyperactive, bowel sounds are associated with ileus.

2. You should consider the bowel sounds absent after listening for how long without hearing any?

    a. 2 minutes

    b. 3 minutes

    c. 4 minutes

    d. 5 minutes

Answer: d. Be sure to allow enough time, about 2 minutes, to listen in each quadrant before deciding that the bowel sounds are absent.

3. Which two percussion sounds are normally heard over the abdomen?

    a. Tympany and dullness

    b. Resonance and tympany

    c. Flatness and dullness

    d. Flatness and hyperresonance

Answer: a. Tympany is heard when percussing over hollow organs, such as an empty stomach. Dullness is heard when percussing over solid organs, such as the liver or feces-filled intestines.

4. If a patient presents with diarrhea, it's essential to monitor his:

    a. blood pressure.

    b. fluid and electrolyte balance.

    c. temperature.

    d. blood glucose level.

Answer: b. The fluid and electrolyte imbalances that diarrhea produces may precipitate life-threatening arrhythmias or hypovolemic shock. The patient's fluid and electrolyte balance should be monitored closely.

5. Abdominal pain can be caused by disorders from which body systems?

    a. GI system

    b. Reproductive system

    c. Musculoskeletal system

    d. All of the above

Answer: d. Because the abdomen houses so many organs, it's important to remember that abdominal pain isn't always caused by a GI disorder.

Musculoskeletal system

When a patient complains of a problem related to the musculoskeletal system, you usually don't have a life-threatening situation—but, at times, you may. A severe injury can lead to blood loss and shock. And a muscle spasm may be the first sign of hypocalcemic tetany.

Typically, your patient's chief sign or symptom will indicate a problem in the bone, muscle, soft-tissue, or neurologic or vascular system. This chapter will help you investigate the source of such signs or symptoms by providing a general review of the anatomy and physiology of the musculoskeletal system, along with essential physical assessment techniques and 3-minute assessment guidelines to help you focus on the patient's chief sign or symptom. (See *Musculoskeletal system: Normal findings,* page 126.)

Anatomy and physiology

The structures of the musculoskeletal system give the human body its shape and ability to move. The three main parts of the musculoskeletal system are the bones, joints, and muscles.

The 206 bones of the skeleton form the body's framework, supporting or-

gans and tissues. The bones also serve as storage sites for minerals and produce blood cells. (See *Structures of the skeletal system,* pages 128 and 129.)

The junction of two or more bones is a joint. Joints stabilize the bones and allow movement.

Skeletal muscles are groups of contractile cells or fibers. These fibers contract and produce skeletal movement when they receive a stimulus from the central nervous system (CNS).

Physical assessment

Because the CNS and the musculoskeletal system are interrelated, you should assess them together.

To assess the musculoskeletal system, use inspection and palpation to test all the major bones, joints, and muscles. Perform a complete examination if the patient has generalized symptoms such as aching in several joints. Perform an abbreviated examination if he has pain in only one body area such as his ankle.

Begin your examination with a general observation of the patient. Then systematically assess the whole body, working from head to toe and from proximal to distal structures. Because muscles and joints are interdependent, interpret these findings together. As

CHECKLIST

Musculoskeletal system: Normal findings

Inspection
❑ No gross deformities are apparent.
❑ Body parts are symmetrical.
❑ Body is in alignment.
❑ No involuntary movements are detectable.
❑ Gait is smooth.
❑ All muscles and joints have active range of motion, with no pain.
❑ No swelling or inflammation is visible in the joints or muscles.

❑ Bilateral limb length is equal, and muscle mass is symmetrical.

Palpation
❑ Shape is normal, with no swelling or tenderness.
❑ Bilateral muscle tone, texture, and strength are equal.
❑ No involuntary contractions or twitching is detectable.
❑ Bilateral pulses are equally strong.

---

you work your way down the body, follow these general rules:

■ Note the size, shape and symmetry of joints, limbs, and body regions.
■ Inspect and palpate the skin and tissues around the joint, limbs, and body regions. Note any masses , deformities, tenderness, or muscle atrophy.
■ Have the patient perform active range-of-motion (ROM) of each joint, if he is able. If he can't, use passive ROM. Compare bilateral joint findings.
■ During passive ROM, support the joint firmly on either side, and move it gently to avoid causing pain or spasm.

Whenever possible, observe his gait and posture, and how the patient stands and moves. Watch him walk into the room or, if he's already in, ask him to walk to the door, turn around, and walk back toward you. The torso should sway only slightly, arms should swing naturally at the sides, gait should be even, and posture should be erect.

As he walks, his foot should flatten and bear his weight completely, and his toes should flex as he pushes off with his foot. In midswing, his foot should clear the floor and pass the other leg.

ASSESSING THE BONES AND JOINTS

Perform a head-to-toe evaluation of your patient's bones and joints using inspection and palpation. Then perform a ROM assessment to help you determine whether the joints are healthy. Do not move any joints past the point of pain. Elderly patients may experience discomfort with some of the positions if they have decreased flexibility.

Head, jaw, and neck

Inspect the patient's face for swelling, symmetry, and evidence of trauma. The mandible should be in the midline, not shifted to the right or left.

Evaluate ROM in the temporomandibular joint. Place the tips of your first two or three fingers in front of the middle of the ear. Ask the patient to open and close his mouth. Then place your fingers into the depressed area over the joint, and note the motion of the mandible. The patient should be able to open and close his jaw and protract and retract his mandible easily, without pain or tenderness. If you hear or palpate a click as the patient's mouth opens, suspect an improperly aligned jaw.

Inspect the front, back, and sides of the patient's neck, noting muscle asymmetry or masses. Palpate the spinous processes of the cervical vertebrae and supraclavicular fossae for tenderness, swelling, or nodules.

To palpate the neck area, stand facing the patient with your hands placed lightly on the sides of the neck. Ask him to turn his head from side to side, flex his neck forward, and then extend it backward. Feel for lumps or tender areas.

As the patient moves his neck, listen and palpate for crepitus. This is an abnormal crunching or grating sound, not the occasional "crack" we hear from our joints.

Now, check ROM in the neck. Ask the patient to try touching his right ear to his right shoulder and left ear to left shoulder. The usual ROM is 40 degrees on each side. Next, ask him to touch his chin to his chest and then to point his chin toward the ceiling. The neck should flex forward 45 degrees and extend backward 55 degrees.

To assess rotation, ask the patient to turn his head to each side without moving his trunk. His chin should be parallel to his shoulders. Finally, ask him to move his head in a circle—normal rotation is 70 degrees.

Spine

Ask the patient to remove his hospital gown so you can observe his spine. First, check spinal curvature as he stands in profile. In this position, the spine has a reverse S shape.

Next, observe the spine posteriorly. It should be in midline position, without deviation to either side. Lateral deviation suggests scoliosis. You also may notice that one shoulder is lower than the other or that the hips are uneven.

To assess the patient for scoliosis, have him bend at the waist. This position makes deformities more apparent. Normally, the spine remains at midline.

Next, assess the ROM of the spine. Ask the patient to straighten up, and use the measuring tape to measure the distance from the nape of his neck to his waist. Then ask him to bend forward at the waist. Continue to hold the tape at his neck, letting it slip through your fingers slightly to accommodate the increased distance as the spine flexes.

The length of the spine from neck to waist usually increases by at least 2″ (5 cm) when the patient bends forward. If it doesn't, the patient's mobility may be impaired, and you'll need to assess him further.

Finally, palpate the spinal processes and the areas lateral to the spine. Have the patient bend at the waist and let his arms hang loosely at his sides. Palpate the spine with your fingertips. Then repeat the palpation using the side of your hand, lightly striking the areas lateral to the spine. Note tenderness, swelling, or spasm.

Shoulders and elbows

Start by observing the patient's shoulders, noting asymmetry, muscle atrophy, or deformity.

Palpate the shoulders with the palmar surfaces of your fingers to locate

(Text continues on page 130.)

Structures of the skeletal system

Of the 206 bones in the human skeletal system, 80 form the axial skeleton, or head and trunk, and 126 form the appendicular skeleton, or the extremities. Shown below are the body's major bones.

Anterior view

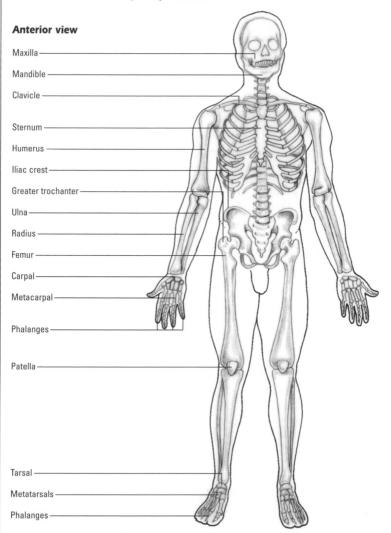

Maxilla

Mandible

Clavicle

Sternum

Humerus

Iliac crest

Greater trochanter

Ulna

Radius

Femur

Carpal

Metacarpal

Phalanges

Patella

Tarsal

Metatarsals

Phalanges

Posterior view

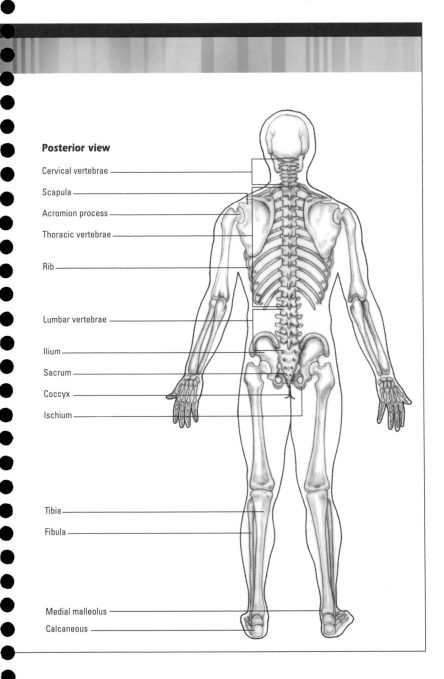

Cervical vertebrae

Scapula

Acromion process

Thoracic vertebrae

Rib

Lumbar vertebrae

Ilium

Sacrum

Coccyx

Ischium

Tibia

Fibula

Medial malleolus

Calcaneous

bony landmarks; note crepitus or tenderness. Using your entire hand, palpate the shoulder muscles for firmness and symmetry. Also palpate the elbow and the ulna for subcutaneous nodules that occur with rheumatoid arthritis.

If the patient tolerates shoulder movement, assess rotation. Start with the patient's arm straight at his side—the neutral position. Ask him to lift his arm straight up from his side to shoulder level and then to bend his elbow horizontally until his forearm is at a 90-degree angle to his upper arm. The arm should be parallel to the floor, and fingers should be extended with palms down.

To assess external rotation, have him bring his forearm up until his fingers point toward the ceiling. To assess internal rotation, have him lower his forearm until his fingers point toward the floor. Normal ROM is 90 degrees in each direction.

To assess flexion and extension, start with the patient's arm in the neutral position (at his side). To assess flexion, ask him to move his arm anteriorly over his head, as if reaching for the sky. Full flexion is 180 degrees. To assess extension, have him move his arm from the neutral position posteriorly as far as possible. Normal extension ranges from 30 to 50 degrees.

To assess abduction, ask the patient to move his arm from the neutral position laterally as far as possible. Normal ROM is 180 degrees.

To assess adduction, have the patient move his arm from the neutral position across the front of his body as far as possible. Normal ROM is 50 degrees.

Next, assess the elbows for flexion and extension. Have the patient rest his arm at his side. Ask him to flex his elbow from this position and then extend it. Normal ROM is 90 degrees for both flexion and extension.

To assess supination and pronation of the elbow, have the patient place the side of his hand on a flat surface with the thumb on top. Ask him to rotate his palm down toward the table for pronation and upward for supination. The normal angle of elbow rotation is 90 degrees in each direction.

Wrists and hands

Inspect the wrists and hands for contour, and compare them for symmetry. Also check for nodules, redness, swelling, deformities, and webbing between fingers.

Use your thumb and index finger to palpate both wrists and each finger joint. Note any tenderness, swelling, nodules, or crepitation. To avoid causing pain, be especially gentle, particularly if the patient is elderly or has arthritis.

Assess ROM in the wrist. Ask the patient to rotate his wrist by moving his entire hand—first laterally then medially—as if he's waxing a car. Normal ROM is 55 degrees laterally and 20 degrees medially.

Observe the wrist while the patient extends his fingers up toward the ceiling and down toward the floor, as if he's flapping his hand. He should be able to extend his wrist 70 degrees and flex it 90 degrees.

To assess extension and flexion of the metacarpophalangeal joints, ask the patient to keep his wrist still and move only his fingers—first up toward the ceiling and down toward the floor. Normal extension is 30 degrees; normal flexion, 90 degrees.

Next, ask the patient to touch his thumb to the little finger of the same hand. He should be able to fold or flex his thumb across the palm of his hand so that it touches or points toward the base of his little finger.

To assess flexion of all of the fingers, ask the patient to form a fist. Then have him spread his fingers apart to demonstrate abduction and draw them back together to demonstrate adduction.

If you suspect that one arm is longer than the other, take measurements. Put one end of the measuring tape at the acromion process of the shoulder and the other on the tip of the middle finger. Drape the tape over the outer elbow. The difference between the left and right extremities should be no more than $3/8"$ (1 cm).

Hips and knees

Inspect the hip area for contour and symmetry. Inspect the position of the knees, noting whether the patient is bowlegged or knock-kneed. Then watch the patient walk.

Palpate both knees. They should feel smooth, and the tissues should feel solid. (See *Bulge sign,* page 132.)

Assess ROM in the hip. If the patient has had a total hip replacement, do not test ROM unless the physician gives permission. Ideally, these exercises should be done with the patient standing. But if he's elderly or if he has trouble standing, he can lie in a supine position instead.

To assess hip flexion, have the patient stand and extend his leg forward. He should be able to move his leg forward between 45 and 90 degrees. To assess hip extension, have him return the leg to a straight position (0 degrees). To assess hyperextension, ask him to extend the leg backward, keeping his knees straight. He should be

able to extend his leg about 30 degrees backward.

Next, have him kick out laterally to assess abduction and swing one leg across the other to assess adduction. Normal ROM is about 45 degrees for abduction and 30 degrees for adduction.

To assess internal and external rotation of the hip, ask the patient to lift one leg up and, keeping his knee straight, turn the leg and foot medially and laterally. Normal ROM for internal rotation is 40 degrees; for external rotation, 45 degrees.

Assess ROM in the knee. If the patient is standing, ask him to bend his knee as if trying to touch his heel to his buttocks. Normal ROM for flexion is 120 to 130 degrees. If the patient is lying down, have him draw his knee up to his chest. His calf should touch his thigh.

Knee extension returns the knee to a neutral position of 0 degrees; however, some knees may normally be hyperextended 15 degrees. If the patient can't extend his leg fully or if his knee "pops" audibly and painfully, consider the response abnormal.

Ankles and feet

Inspect the ankles and feet for swelling, redness, nodules, and other deformities. Check the arch of the foot and look for toe deformities. Also note edema, calluses, bunions, corns, ingrown toenails, plantar warts, trophic ulcers, hair loss, or unusual pigmentation.

Use your fingertips to palpate the bony and muscular structures of the ankles and feet. Palpate each toe joint by compressing it with your thumb and fingers.

Bulge sign

The bulge sign indicates excess fluid in the joint. To assess the patient for this sign, ask him to lie down so that you can palpate his knee. Then give the medial side of his knee two to four firm strokes, as shown, to displace excess fluid.

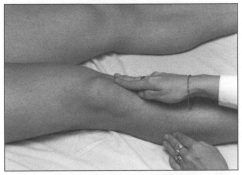

Lateral check
Next, tap the lateral aspect of the knee while checking for a fluid wave on the medial aspect, as shown.

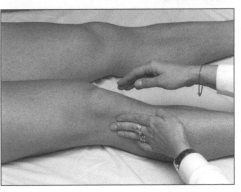

To examine the ankle, have the patient sit in a chair or on the side of a bed. To test plantar flexion, ask him to point his toes toward the floor. Test dorsiflexion by asking him to point his toes toward the ceiling. Normal ROM for plantar flexion is about 45 degrees; for dorsiflexion, 20 degrees.

Next, assess ROM in the ankle. Ask the patient to demonstrate inversion by turning his feet inward and eversion by turning his feet outward. Normal ROM for inversion is 45 degrees; for eversion, 30 degrees.

To assess the metatarsophalangeal joints, ask the patient to flex his toes and then straighten them.

If you suspect that one leg is longer than the other, take measurements. Put one end of the tape at the medial malleolus at the ankle and the other end at the anterior iliac spine. Cross the tape over the medial side of the knee. A difference of more than 3/8" (1 cm) is abnormal.

ASSESSING THE MUSCLES

Start by inspecting all major muscle groups for tone, strength, asymmetry, and other abnormalities. If a muscle appears atrophied or hypertrophied, measure it by wrapping a tape measure around the largest circumference of the muscle on each side of the body and comparing the two numbers.

Muscle tone describes muscular resistance to passive stretching. To test the patient's arm muscle tone, move his shoulder through passive ROM. You should feel a slight resistance. Then let the arm drop. It should fall easily to his side.

Test leg muscle tone by putting the patient's hip through passive ROM and then letting the leg fall to the examination table or bed. Like the arm, the leg should fall easily.

Observe the patient's gait and movements to form an idea of general muscle strength. To test specific muscle groups, ask him to move the muscles while you apply resistance; then compare the contralateral muscle groups.

Grade muscle strength on a scale of 0 to 5, with 0 representing no strength and 5 representing maximum strength. Document the results as a fraction, with the score as the numerator and maximum strength as the denominator. (See *Grading muscle strength*.)

Shoulder, arm, wrist, and hand strength

Test the strength of the patient's shoulder girdle by asking him to extend his arms with the palms up and hold this position for 30 seconds. If he can't lift both arms equally and keep his palms up, or if one arm drifts down, he proba-

> ### Grading muscle strength
>
> Grade muscle strength on a scale of 0 to 5, as follows:
> - 5/5: normal; patient moves joint through full range of motion (ROM) and against gravity with full resistance
> - 4/5: good; patient completes ROM against gravity with moderate resistance
> - 3/5: fair; patient completes ROM against gravity only
> - 2/5: poor; patient completes full ROM with gravity eliminated (passive motion)
> - 1/5: trace; patient's attempt at muscle contraction is palpable but without joint movement
> - 0/5: zero; no evidence of muscle contraction.

bly has shoulder girdle weakness on that side.

If he passes the first part of the test, gauge strength by lacing your hands on his arms and applying downward pressure as he resists you.

Next, have the patient hold his arm in front of him with the elbow bent. To test biceps strength, pull down on the flexor surface of his forearm as he resists. To test triceps strength, have him try to straighten his arm as you push upward against the extensor surface of his forearm.

Assess the strength of the patient's flexed wrist by pushing against it. Test the strength of the extended wrist by pushing down on it. Test the strength of finger abduction, thumb opposition, and handgrip the same way.

Age-related changes in elderly people

Musculoskeletal changes continue throughout the adult years. An elderly patient may experience any of these normal musculoskeletal system changes.

• Loss of bone mass and bone strength caused by osteoporosis and decreased exercise
• Joint stiffness and swelling caused by joint degeneration
• Decreased mobility, range of motion, and flexibility
• Decrease in height because of thinning and drying of the intervertebral bodies, which shorten or even collapse
• Muscle atrophy and decrease in muscle strength caused by muscle fiber degeneration, decrease in exercise or activity, and some systemic diseases (should be bilateral if related to aging)
• Deformities in joints: arthritic changes including bow-legged appearance or kyphosis
• Impaired sense of space, which may affect balance or gait and increase risk of falls
• Shrunk and sclerosed tendons, which may result in more muscle cramping

Leg strength

Ask the patient to lie in a supine position on the examination table or bed and have him lift both legs at the same time. Note whether he lifts both legs at the same time and to the same distance. To test quadriceps strength, have him lower his legs and raise them again while you press down on his anterior thighs.

Then ask the patient to flex his knees and put his feet flat on the bed. Assess lower-leg strength by pulling his lower leg forward as he resists and then by pushing it backward as he extends his knee.

Finally, assess ankle strength by having the patient push his foot down against your resistance and then pull his foot up as you try to hold it down. (See *Age-related changes in elderly people.*)

Guidelines for a 3-minute assessment

A 3-minute assessment of signs or symptoms relating to the musculoskeletal system includes making general observations, checking the patient's vital signs, and focusing on the patient's chief sign or symptom. You'll perform this assessment if your patient reports having a problem with his arm or leg or if you suspect he has injured a limb.

MAKING GENERAL OBSERVATIONS

Your general observations of the patient include checking level of consciousness, overall appearance, and skin color.

Level of consciousness

Note whether the patient seems anxious or restless. You may see these signs of shock if the patient has significant blood loss from a limb injury.

Overall appearance

Observe your patient's overall appearance, including posture. Note obvious injuries or deformities of the limbs. Look for muscle atrophy, and note whether the limbs are symmetrical.

Skin color

Note changes in skin color, such as pallor or mottling, which may indicate peripheral hypoperfusion and shock. Depending on the patient's normal skin color, pallor may be difficult to see. In a light-skinned patient, it may be just a subtle lightening of the skin. With a dark-skinned patient, you may need to check his nail beds.

Increased redness, accompanied by heat, may indicate infection or inflammation. Obvious discoloration—such as petechiae, bruising, or ecchymoses—or breaks in skin integrity indicate injury. Also, look for lesions, visible masses, and areas of swelling or bleeding.

CHECKING VITAL SIGNS

Take your patient's vital signs and compare them with baseline measurements. His pulse rate and blood pressure will give you a good indication of blood flow in the limbs. A fall in systolic blood pressure to 80 mm Hg, or 30 mm Hg less than the patient's baseline, accompanied by a narrowing pulse pressure and a rapid, weak and, in many cases, irregular pulse may indicate hypovolemic shock.

Unless you suspect infection, you won't need to take a patient's temperature.

FOCUSING ON THE CHIEF SIGN OR SYMPTOM

After you've made general observations and checked the patient's vital signs, you'll want to focus on the patient's chief musculoskeletal sign or symptom for the history and physical assessment.

Further assessment

As mentioned, you may need to assess another part of the body. For example, if your patient has motor problems, you may also need to evaluate sensory function with a neurologic assessment. (See *Musculoskeletal system: Interpreting your findings,* pages 136 to 138.)

Common signs and symptoms

A patient may seek care for any of a number of signs and symptoms related to the musculoskeletal system. Some common ones are arm pain, leg pain, muscle spasms, and muscle weakness. The following history and physical assessment tips will help you assess each one quickly and accurately.

(Text continues on page 138.)

Musculoskeletal system: Interpreting your findings

After you assess the patient, a group of findings may lead you to suspect a particular disorder. The chart below shows some common groups of findings for signs and symptoms of the musculoskeletal system, along with their probable causes.

Sign or symptom and findings	Probable cause
Arm pain	
• Pain radiating through the arm • Pain worsens with movement • Crepitus, felt and heard • Deformity (if bones are misaligned) • Local ecchymosis and edema • Impaired distal circulation • Paresthesia	Fracture
• Left arm pain • Deep and crushing chest pain • Weakness • Pallor • Dyspnea • Diaphoresis • Apprehension	Myocardial infarction
• Severe arm pain with passive muscle stretching • Impaired distal circulation • Muscle weakness • Decreased reflex response • Paresthesia • Edema • Ominous signs: paralysis and absent pulse	Compartment syndrome
Leg pain	
• Severe, acute leg pain, particularly with movement • Ecchymosis and edema • Leg unable to bear weight • Impaired neurovascular status distal to injury • Deformity, crepitus, and muscle spasms	Fracture

Musculoskeletal system: Interpreting your findings
(continued)

Sign or symptom and findings	Probable cause
Leg pain *(continued)*	
• Shooting, aching, or tingling pain that radiates down the leg • Pain exacerbated by activity and relieved by rest • Limping • Difficulty moving from a sitting to a standing position	Sciatica
• Discomfort ranging from calf tenderness to severe pain • Edema and a feeling of heaviness in the affected leg • Warmth • Fever, chills, malaise, muscle cramps • Positive Homan's sign	Thrombophlebitis
• Deep, aching joint pain • Crepitation in joint area • Enlarged edematous joint with deformities • Joint stiffness • Decreased range of motion • Heberden's nodes	Osteoarthritis
Muscle spasm	
• Spasms and intermittent claudication • Loss of peripheral pulses • Pallor or cyanosis • Decreased sensation • Hair loss • Dry or scaling skin • Edema • Ulcerations	Arterial occlusive disease
• Localized spasms and pain • Swelling • Limited mobility • Bony crepitation	Fracture
• Tetany (muscle cramps and twitching, carpopedal and facial muscle spasms, and seizures) • Positive Chvostek's and Trousseau's signs • Paresthesia of the lips, fingers, and toes	Hypocalcemia

(continued)

Musculoskeletal system: Interpreting your findings
(continued)

Sign or symptom and findings	Probable cause
Muscle spasm (continued)	
• Choreiform movements • Hyperactive deep tendon reflexes • Fatigue • Palpitations • Cardiac arrhythmias	Hypocalcemia (continued)
Muscle weakness	
• Unilateral or bilateral weakness of the arms, legs, face, or tongue • Dysarthria • Aphasia • Paresthesia or sensory loss • Vision disturbances • Bowel and bladder dysfunction	Stroke
• Muscle weakness, disuse, and possible atrophy • Altered level of consciousness • Personality changes • Severe low back pain, possibly radiating to the buttocks, legs, and feet (usually unilateral) • Diminished reflexes • Sensory changes	Herniated disk
• Muscle weakness in one or more limbs which may lead to atrophy, spasticity, and contractures • Diplopia, blurred vision, or vision loss • Hyperactive deep tendon reflexes • Paresthesia or sensory loss • Incoordination • Intention tremors	Multiple sclerosis

MUSCLE SPASMS

Muscle spasms, or cramps, are strong, painful contractions. They can occur in virtually any muscle but are most common in the calf and foot.

History

If the patient isn't in distress, ask when the spasms began. How long did they last? How painful were they? Did anything worsen or lessen the pain? Ask about other symptoms, such as weakness, sensory loss, or paresthesia.

Physical assessment

Evaluate muscle strength and tone. Then check all major muscle groups, and note whether any movements precipitate spasms. Test the presence and quality of all peripheral pulses, and examine the limbs for color and temperature changes. Test capillary refill time, and inspect for edema, especially in the involved area. Finally, test reflexes and sensory function in all extremities.

Analysis
Muscle spasms typically occur with simple muscle fatigue, after exercise, and during pregnancy. However, they may also result from an electrolyte imbalance, such as hypocalcemia; a neuromuscular disorder; or use of certain drugs. They're typically precipitated by movement, and they can usually be relieved by slow stretching.

PEDIATRIC TIP
Muscle spasms rarely occur in children. However, their presence may indicate hypoparathyroidism, osteomalacia, rickets or, rarely, congenital torticollis.

MUSCLE WEAKNESS
Muscle weakness may be reported to you by the patient, or it may be something you detect by observing and measuring the strength of an individual muscle or muscle group.

History
Begin by determining the location of the patient's muscle weakness. Ask if he has difficulty with specific movements, such as rising from a chair. Find out when he first noticed the weakness; ask him whether it worsens with exercise or as the day progresses. Ask about related symptoms, especially muscle or joint pain, altered sensory function, and fatigue.

Obtain a medical history, noting especially chronic disease, such as hyperthyroidism; musculoskeletal or neurologic problems, including recent trauma; family history of chronic muscle weakness, especially in men; and use of alcohol or certain drugs.

Physical assessment
Focus your physical examination on evaluating muscle strength. Test all major muscles bilaterally. When testing, make sure the patient's effort is constant; if it isn't, suspect pain or other reluctance to make the effort. If the patient complains of pain, ease or discontinue testing, and have him try the movements again. Remember that the patient's dominant arm, hand, and leg are somewhat stronger than their nondominant counterparts. Besides testing individual muscle strength, test the ROM at all major joints, including the shoulder, elbow, wrist, hip, knee, and ankle. Also test sensory function in the involved areas, and test deep tendon reflexes bilaterally.

Analysis
Muscle weakness can result from a malfunction in the cerebral hemispheres, brain stem, spinal cord, nerve roots, peripheral nerves, or myoneural junctions and within the muscle itself. Muscle weakness occurs in certain neurologic, musculoskeletal, metabolic, endocrine, and cardiovascular disorders; as a response to certain drugs; and after prolonged immobilization.

PEDIATRIC TIP
Muscular dystrophy, usually the Duchenne type, is a major cause of muscle weakness in children.

Elderly patients may have decreased muscle strength due to muscle fiber degeneration.

ARM PAIN

Arm pain usually results from musculoskeletal disorders, but it can also stem from neurovascular or cardiovascular disorders. In some cases, it may be referred pain from another area, such as the chest, neck, or abdomen.

History

If the patient reports arm pain after an injury, take a brief history of the injury. Then quickly assess him for severe injuries requiring immediate treatment. If you've ruled out severe injuries, check pulses, capillary refill time, sensation, and movement distal to the affected area because circulatory impairment or nerve injury may require immediate surgery. Inspect the arm for deformities, assess the level of pain, and immobilize the arm to prevent further injury.

If the patient reports continuous or intermittent arm pain, ask him to describe it and relate when it began. Is the pain associated with repetitive or specific movements or positions? Ask him to point out other painful areas because arm pain may be referred. For example, arm pain commonly accompanies the characteristic chest pain of myocardial infarction, and right shoulder pain may be referred from the right upper quadrant abdominal pain of cholecystitis. Ask the patient if the pain worsens in the morning or in the evening, if it prevents him from performing his job, and if it restricts movement. Also ask if heat, rest, or drugs relieve it. Finally, ask about any preexisting illnesses, a family history

of gout or arthritis, and current drug therapy.

Physical assessment

Next, perform a focused examination. Observe the way the patient walks, sits, and holds his arm. Inspect the entire arm, comparing it with the opposite arm for symmetry, movement, and muscle atrophy. (It's important to know whether the patient is right- or left-handed.) Palpate the entire arm for swelling, nodules, and tender areas. In both arms, compare active ROM, muscle strength, and reflexes.

If the patient reports numbness or tingling, check his sensation to vibration, temperature, and pinprick. Compare bilateral hand grasps and shoulder strength to detect weakness.

If a patient has a cast, splint, or restrictive dressing, check for circulation, sensation, and mobility distal to the dressing. Ask him if he has experienced edema and if the pain has worsened within the last 24 hours. Also ask which activities he has been performing.

Examine the neck for pain on motion, point tenderness, muscle spasms, or arm pain when the neck is extended with the head toward the involved side.

Analysis

The location, onset, and character of the arm pain provide clues to its cause. The pain may affect the entire arm or only the upper arm or forearm. It may occur suddenly or gradually and be constant or intermittent. Arm pain can be described as sharp or dull, burning or numbing, and shooting or penetrating. Diffuse arm pain, though, may be difficult to describe, especially if it isn't associated with injury.

In children, arm pain commonly results from fractures, muscle sprain, muscular dystrophy, or rheumatoid arthritis. In young children especially, the exact location of the pain may be difficult to establish. Watch for nonverbal clues, such as wincing or guarding.

If the child has a fracture or sprain, obtain a complete account of the injury. Closely observe interactions between the child and his family, and don't rule out the possibility of child abuse.

GERIATRIC TIP

Elderly patients with osteoporosis may experience fractures from simple trauma or even from heavy lifting or unexpected movements. They're also prone to degenerative joint disease that can involve several joints in the arm or neck.

LEG PAIN

Although leg pain often signifies a musculoskeletal disorder, it can also result from more serious vascular or neurologic disorders. The pain may occur suddenly or gradually and may be localized or affect the entire leg. Constant or intermittent, it may feel dull, burning, sharp, shooting, or tingling.

History

If the patient's condition permits, ask him when the pain began and have him describe its intensity, character, and pattern. Is the pain worse in the morning, at night, or with movement? If it doesn't prevent him from walking, must he rely on a crutch or other assistive device? Also, ask him about the presence of other signs and symptoms.

Find out if the patient has a history of leg injury or surgery, and if he or a family member has a history of joint, vascular, or back problems. Also, ask what medications he's taking and whether they've helped to relieve leg pain.

Physical assessment

Begin the physical examination by watching the patient walk, if his condition permits. Observe how he holds his leg while standing and sitting. Palpate the legs, buttocks, and lower back to determine the extent of pain and tenderness. If fracture has been ruled out, test ROM in the hip and knee. Also, check reflexes with the patient's leg straightened and raised, noting any action that causes pain. Then compare both legs for symmetry, movement, and active ROM. Also, assess sensation and strength. If the patient wears a leg cast, splint, or restrictive dressing, carefully check distal circulation, sensation, and mobility, and stretch his toes to elicit any associated pain.

Analysis

Leg pain typically affects movement, limiting weight bearing. Severe leg pain that follows cast application for a fracture may signal limb-threatening compartment syndrome. Sudden onset of severe leg pain in a patient with underlying vascular insufficiency may signal acute deterioration, possibly requiring an arterial graft or amputation.

PEDIATRIC TIP

Common pediatric causes of leg pain include fracture, osteomyelitis, and bone cancer. If parents fail to give an adequate explanation for a leg fracture, consider the possibility of child abuse.

Leg pain may also be normal in children during growth periods. It's important to differentiate when children complain of leg pain.

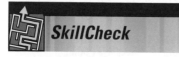

SkillCheck

1. The bulge sign should be used to test which physical finding?
    a. A swollen knee
    b. A swollen ankle
    c. A swollen hand
    d. A swollen elbow
Answer: a. The bulge sign is used to evaluate fluid in the knee.

2. In a patient with scoliosis, you *would* find:
    a. midline position of the spine.
    b. even hip height.
    c. uneven shoulder height.
    d. abnormally concave lumbar spine.
Answer: c. A patient with scoliosis often has uneven shoulder height.

3. If a patient comes into your facility with muscle weakness, where should you focus your physical assessment?
    a. Muscle tone
    b. Muscle strength
    c. ROM
    d. Sensory function
Answer: b. Although your assessment may include checking all of these areas, the essential component of your assessment should be checking the muscle strength of all major muscles bilaterally.

4. A patient comes into your facility with severe pain, swelling, and bruising in the right leg and is unable to bear weight on that leg. His extremity is cool to touch below the injury. You suspect:
    a. sciatica.
    b. strain.
    c. sprain.
    d. fracture.
Answer: d. You should think of a fracture, especially if movement causes extreme pain.

5. Which assessment technique gives important clues about the patient's bones, muscles, and joints?
    a. Watching the patient walk
    b. Palpating the skin around the joint
    c. Having the patient bend at the waist
    d. Checking reflexes
Answer: a. Watching the patient walk can give you important clues about bones, muscles, and joints and may guide the rest of your physical assessment. If he's limping, one leg may be longer than the other, or he may have an injury in one leg.

Integumentary system

The skin covers the internal structures of the body and protects them from the external world. Along with hair and nails, the skin provides a window for viewing changes taking place inside the body and for detecting abnormalities. Your sharp assessment skills will help supply a reliable picture of the patient's overall health.

This chapter will help you do a quick and accurate assessment of the integumentary system by reviewing anatomy and physiology, physical assessment techniques, and guidelines for a 3-minute assessment of signs and symptoms related to the skin, hair, and nails.

Anatomy and physiology

The integumentary system consists of the skin and anything attached to it, such as the hair and nails.

SKIN

The skin is the body's largest organ and has several important functions, including:

- protecting underlying tissues from trauma and bacteria and preventing the loss of water and electrolytes from the body

- sensing temperature, pain, touch, and pressure
- regulating body temperature through sweat production and evaporation
- synthesizing vitamin D
- promoting wound repair by allowing cell replacement of surface wounds.

The skin consists of two distinct layers: the epidermis and the dermis. Subcutaneous tissue lies beneath these layers. (See *Structures of the skin,* page 144.) The epidermis—the outer layer—is made of squamous epithelial tissue. The two major layers of the epidermis are the stratum corneum, which is the most superficial layer, and the deeper basal cell layer, or stratum germinativum.

The dermis—the thick, deeper layer—consists of connective tissue and an extracellular material called matrix, which contributes to the skin's strength and pliability. Blood vessels, lymphatic vessels, nerves, and hair follicles are located in the dermis as well as sweat and sebaceous glands. Wound healing and infection control take place in the dermis.

HAIR

Hair is formed from keratin and produced by matrix cells in the dermal layer. Each hair lies in a hair follicle and receives nourishment from the papilla, a loop of capillaries at the base of the follicle. At the lower end of the

Structures of the skin

This cross section of the skin illustrates major skin structures.

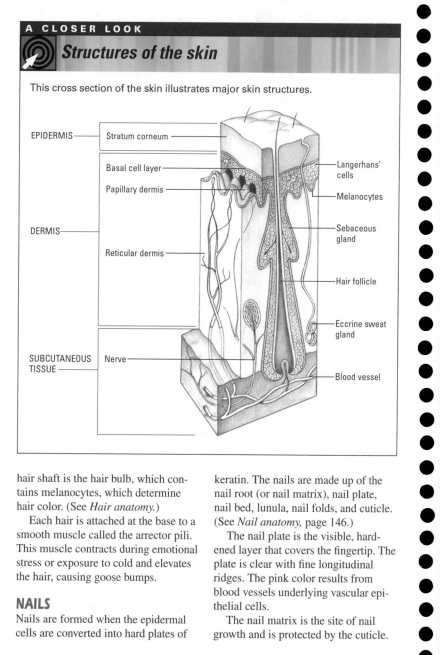

EPIDERMIS — Stratum corneum

Basal cell layer
Papillary dermis

DERMIS

Reticular dermis

SUBCUTANEOUS
TISSUE — Nerve

Langerhans'
cells

Melanocytes

Sebaceous
gland

Hair follicle

Eccrine sweat
gland

Blood vessel

hair shaft is the hair bulb, which contains melanocytes, which determine hair color. (See *Hair anatomy.*)

Each hair is attached at the base to a smooth muscle called the arrector pili. This muscle contracts during emotional stress or exposure to cold and elevates the hair, causing goose bumps.

NAILS

Nails are formed when the epidermal cells are converted into hard plates of keratin. The nails are made up of the nail root (or nail matrix), nail plate, nail bed, lunula, nail folds, and cuticle. (See *Nail anatomy,* page 146.)

The nail plate is the visible, hardened layer that covers the fingertip. The plate is clear with fine longitudinal ridges. The pink color results from blood vessels underlying vascular epithelial cells.

The nail matrix is the site of nail growth and is protected by the cuticle.

Hair anatomy

The illustration below shows a hair shaft and its associated glands.

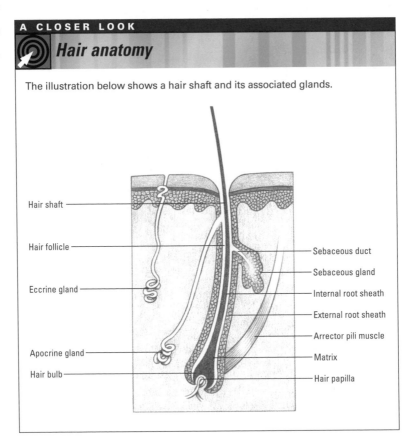

Hair shaft

Hair follicle

Eccrine gland

Apocrine gland

Hair bulb

Sebaceous duct

Sebaceous gland

Internal root sheath

External root sheath

Arrector pili muscle

Matrix

Hair papilla

At the end of the matrix is the white, crescent-shaped area, the lunula, that extends beyond the cuticle.

Physical assessment

To assess skin, hair, and nails, you'll use inspection and palpation. Before beginning the examination, make sure the room is well lit and comfortably warm, and put on gloves. Assess pa-

tient for latex sensitivity or allergy. (See *Integumentary system: Normal findings,* page 147.) Keep in mind during your assessment that a nonjudgmental and sensitive approach is needed. Some skin disorders are highly visible and affect the patient's body image and self-esteem.

ASSESSING THE SKIN

Before you begin the skin assessment, gather the following equipment: clear centimeter ruler, tongue blade, penlight

A CLOSER LOOK

Nail anatomy

The illustration below shows the anatomic components of a fingernail.

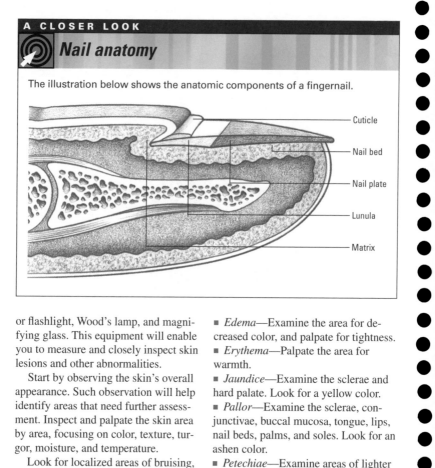

- Cuticle
- Nail bed
- Nail plate
- Lunula
- Matrix

or flashlight, Wood's lamp, and magnifying glass. This equipment will enable you to measure and closely inspect skin lesions and other abnormalities.

Start by observing the skin's overall appearance. Such observation will help identify areas that need further assessment. Inspect and palpate the skin area by area, focusing on color, texture, turgor, moisture, and temperature.

Look for localized areas of bruising, cyanosis, pallor, and erythema. Check for uniformity of color and hypopigmented or hyperpigmented areas. Places exposed to the sun may show a darker pigmentation than other areas. Color changes may vary depending on skin pigmentation. To detect color variations in dark-skinned people, follow these tips:

- *Cyanosis*—Examine the conjunctivae, palms, soles, buccal mucosa, and tongue. Look for dull, dark color.

- *Edema*—Examine the area for decreased color, and palpate for tightness.
- *Erythema*—Palpate the area for warmth.
- *Jaundice*—Examine the sclerae and hard palate. Look for a yellow color.
- *Pallor*—Examine the sclerae, conjunctivae, buccal mucosa, tongue, lips, nail beds, palms, and soles. Look for an ashen color.
- *Petechiae*—Examine areas of lighter pigmentation such as the abdomen. Look for tiny, purplish red dots.
- *Rashes*—Palpate the area for skin texture changes.

Inspect and palpate the skin's texture, noting its thickness and mobility. It should look smooth and be intact. Rough, dry skin is common in patients with hypothyroidism, psoriasis, or excessive keratinization. Skin that isn't intact may indicate local irritation or trauma.

CHECKLIST

Integumentary system: Normal findings

Inspection
❑ Skin color is pink, with no areas of pallor, jaundice, or cyanosis.
❑ No bruising, erythema, or areas of discoloration are apparent.
❑ Skin texture looks smooth and intact.
❑ Normal variations in pigmentation—such as birthmarks, freckles, and nevi—exist.
❑ Quantity and distribution of head and body hair may vary, but it's evenly distributed over the entire body.
❑ No areas of patchy hair loss or excessive hair growth are detectable.

❑ Nail bed color ranges from pink to brown, depending on skin color.
❑ Nail bed is slightly curved or flat.
❑ Nail edges are smooth, rounded, and clean.
❑ Angle of the nail base is 160 degrees or less.

Palpation
❑ Skin feels smooth and warm, without roughened, thickened, or broken areas.
❑ Skin is relatively dry, without excessive perspiration or red, flaky areas.
❑ Skin quickly returns to its original shape when gently squeezed.
❑ Hair is shiny and smooth.

Palpation will also help you evaluate the patient's hydration status. Dehydration and edema cause poor skin turgor. Aging also causes poor skin turgor, so it may not be a reliable indication of fluid status in the elderly. Overhydration causes the skin to appear edematous and spongy. Localized edema can also result from trauma or systemic disease. (See *Evaluating skin turgor,* page 148.)

Observe the skin's moisture content. The skin should be relatively dry, with a minimal amount of perspiration. Skin-fold areas should also be fairly dry. Overly dry skin looks red and flaky. Overly moist skin can be caused by anxiety, obesity, or an environment that's too warm. Diaphoresis usually accompanies fever, strenuous activity, cardiac and pulmonary diseases, and any activity or illness that elevates the metabolic rate.

Palpate the skin for temperature, which can range from cool to warm. Warm skin suggests normal circulation; cool skin, a possible underlying disorder. Distinguish between generalized and localized coolness and warmth. Localized skin coolness can result from vasoconstriction associated with cold environments or impaired arterial circulation to a limb. General coolness can result from such conditions as shock or hypothyroidism.

Localized warmth occurs in areas of infection, inflammation, or burn. Generalized warmth occurs with fever or systemic diseases such as hyperthyroidism. Make sure you check skin temperature bilaterally.

When you're trying to compare subtle temperature differences in one area of the body to another, use the dorsal surface of your hands and fingers. They're the most sensitive to changes in temperature.

Evaluating skin turgor

To assess skin turgor in an adult, gently squeeze the skin on the forearm or sternal area between your thumb and forefinger as shown. In an infant, roll a fold of loosely adherent abdominal skin between your thumb and forefinger. Then release the skin.

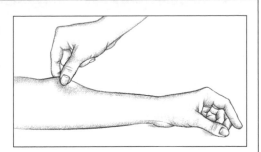

If the skin quickly returns to its original shape, the patient has normal turgor. If it returns to its original shape slowly over 30 seconds, or maintains a tented position as shown, the skin has poor turgor.

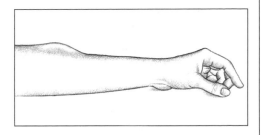

Skin lesions

During your inspection, you may see normal variations in the skin's texture and pigmentation. Red, pigmented lesions caused by vascular changes include hemangiomas, telangiectases, petechiae, purpura, and ecchymoses and may indicate disease.

Other normal variations include birthmarks, freckles, and nevi. Birthmarks are generally flat and range in color from tan to red or brown; they can be found on all areas of the body. Freckles are small, flat macules located primarily on the face, arms, and back and are usually red-brown to brown. Nevi are either flat or raised and may be pink, tan, or dark brown; like birthmarks, they can be found on all areas of the body.

Whenever you see a lesion, evaluate it to determine its origin. Start by classifying it as primary or secondary. A primary lesion is the initial lesion that develops. Changes in a primary lesion then constitute a secondary lesion. Examples of secondary lesions include fissures, scales, crusts, scars, and excoriations. (See *Identifying primary lesions.*)

Determine whether the lesion is solid or fluid filled. Macules, papules, nodules, wheals, and hives are solid lesions. Vesicles, bullae, pustules, and cysts are fluid-filled lesions.

Illuminating a lesion with a flashlight or penlight will help you see it better and learn more about its characteristics. The following two techniques will help you determine what type of

Identifying primary lesions

Primary lesions are typically classified as macules, papules, or vesicles. Here's a quick look at each type. Remember to keep a centimeter ruler handy to accurately measure the lesion's size.

Macule	**Papule**	**Vesicle**
A flat circumscribed area of altered skin color; generally less than ⅜". *Examples:* freckle or flat nevus.	Raised, circumscribed, solid area; generally less than ⅜". *Examples:* elevated nevus or wart.	Circumscribed, elevated lesion; contains serous fluid; less than ⅜". *Example:* early chickenpox.

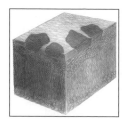 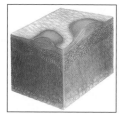 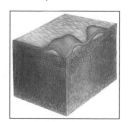

lesion you're dealing with and whether it's solid or fluid-filled:
- To determine whether a lesion is a macule or a papule, reduce the direct lighting and shine a penlight or flashlight at a right angle to the lesion. If the light casts a shadow, the lesion is a papule. Macules are flat and don't produce shadows.
- To determine whether a lesion is solid or fluid-filled, place the tip of a flashlight or penlight against the side of the lesion. Solid lesions don't transmit light. Fluid-filled lesions transilluminate with a red glow.

To identify lesions that fluoresce, use a Wood's lamp, which gives out specially filtered ultraviolet light. Darken the room, and shine the light on the lesion. If the lesion looks bluish green, the patient has a fungal infection.

After you've identified the type of lesion it is, describe its characteristics, pattern, location, and distribution. A detailed description will help you determine whether the lesion is a normal or pathologic skin change.

Examine the lesion to see if it looks the same on both sides. Also, check the borders to see if they're regular or irregular. An asymmetrical lesion with an irregular border may indicate malignancy.

Lesions occur in various colors and can change over time. Therefore, watch for such changes in your patient. For example, if a lesion has changed from tan or brown to multiple shades of tan, dark brown, black, or a mixture of red, white, and blue, the lesion might be malignant. Also, pay close attention to the configuration and distribution of the lesion.

Measure the exact diameter of the lesion using a centimeter ruler. If you estimate the diameter, you may not be able to determine subtle changes in size. An increase in the size or elevation of a mole over a period of many years is common and probably normal. Still, be sure to note moles that change size rapidly.

If you note drainage, document the type, color, and amount. Also, note if the lesion has a foul odor, which can indicate a superimposed infection.

ASSESSING THE HAIR

Start by inspecting and palpating the hair over the patient's entire body, not just on his head. Note the distribution, quantity, texture, and color. The quantity and distribution of head and body hair varies among patients. However, hair should be evenly distributed over the entire body.

Check for patterns of hair loss and growth. If you notice patchy hair loss, look for regrowth. Also, examine the scalp for erythema, scaling, and encrustation. Excessive hair loss with scalp crusting may indicate ringworm infestation. The only way to detect scalp crusting is by using a Wood's lamp. Also, note areas of excessive hair growth, which may indicate a hormone imbalance or be a sign of a systemic disorder such as Cushing's syndrome.

The texture of scalp hair also varies among patients. As a rule, hair should be shiny and smooth, not dry or brittle. Differences in grooming and hairstyling may affect the hair's texture and quality. Dryness or brittleness can result from the use of harsh hair treatments or hair care products, or it might be caused by a systemic illness. Extreme oiliness is usually related to an excessive production of sebum or poor grooming habits.

ASSESSING THE NAILS

Assessing the nails is vital for two reasons: The appearance of nails can be a critical indicator of systemic illness, and their overall condition tells you a lot about the patient's grooming habits and ability to care for himself. Examine the nails for color, shape, thickness, consistency, and contour.

First, look at the color of the nails. Light-skinned people generally have pinkish nails. Dark-skinned people generally have brown nails. Brown-pigmented bands in the nail beds are normal in dark-skinned people and abnormal in light-skinned people. Yellow nails may occur in smokers as a result of nicotine stains.

Nail beds can be used to assess a patient's peripheral circulation. Press on the nail bed and then release, noting how long the color takes to return. It should return within 3 seconds.

Next inspect the shape and contour of the nails. The surface of the nail bed should be either slightly curved or flat. The edges of the nail should be smooth, rounded, and clean.

The normal angle of the nail base is 160 degrees. An increase in the nail angle suggests clubbing. Curved nails are a normal variation. They may appear to be clubbed until you notice that the nail angle is still 160 degrees or less.

Finally, palpate the nail bed to check the thickness of the nail and the strength of its attachment to the bed.

Guidelines for a 3-minute assessment

You'll perform a 3-minute assessment of the integumentary system if you note an abnormality or change in the patient's skin, hair, or nail condition or if your patient is experiencing a specific related sign or symptom. Because the skin, hair, and nails indicate what's taking place internally, your findings may suggest a range of problems, from localized injuries to systemic disorders. Begin your assessment by making general observations and taking the patient's vital signs.

MAKING GENERAL OBSERVATIONS

Your general observations of the patient include noting overall appearance and skin condition.

Overall appearance

Note the patient's general hair distribution and nail condition. Hair loss—although it's a normal part of aging—can also result from infection, chemical trauma, ingestion of certain drugs, and endocrinopathy. Excessive hairiness can result from certain drug therapies or an endocrine disorder. Although many nail abnormalities are harmless, some point to serious underlying problems, such as respiratory or cardiovascular disease.

Skin condition

Note changes in skin color, such as pallor or mottling, which may indicate peripheral hypoperfusion or shock. Depending on the patient's normal skin color, pallor can be hard to see, so you may need to check his nail beds. Increased redness, accompanied by heat, may indicate infection or inflammation. Obvious discoloration, such as petechiae, bruising, or ecchymoses or breaks in skin integrity, indicate injury. Also, look for lesions, visible masses, and areas of swelling or bleeding.

CHECKING VITAL SIGNS

Take your patient's vital signs, and compare them with baseline measurements. His pulse rate and blood pressure will give you a good indication of blood flow to the skin.

If the patient feels excessively warm or cool, take his temperature.

FOCUSING ON THE CHIEF SIGN OR SYMPTOM

After you've made general observations and checked the patient's vital signs, you'll want to focus on the patient's chief integumentary sign or symptom for the history and physical assessment.

Further assessment

Even if a patient comes into your facility with integumentary signs or symptoms, you may still need to assess other body systems—such as the respiratory, cardiovascular, or musculoskeletal system—because the problem may be rooted there. (See *Integumentary system: Interpreting your findings*.)

 ## *Integumentary system: Interpreting your findings*

After you assess the patient, a group of findings may lead you to suspect a particular disorder. The chart below shows common groups of findings for the signs and symptoms of the integumentary system, along with their probable causes.

Sign or symptom and findings	Probable cause
Alopecia	
• Patchy alopecia, typically on the lower extremities • Thin, shiny, atrophic skin • Thickened nails • Weak or absent peripheral pulses • Cool extremities • Paresthesia	Arterial insufficiency
• Translucent, charred, or ulcerated skin • Pain	Burns
• Loss of the outer third of the eyebrows • Thin, dull, coarse, brittle hair on the face, scalp, and genitals • Fatigue • Constipation • Cold intolerance • Weight gain • Puffy face, hands, and feet	Hypothyroidism
Clubbing	
• Anorexia • Malaise • Dyspnea • Tachypnea • Diminished breath sounds • Pursed-lip breathing • Barrel chest • Peripheral cyanosis	Emphysema

Integumentary system: Interpreting your findings
(continued)

Sign or symptom and findings	Probable cause
Clubbing (continued)	
• Wheezing • Dyspnea • Fatigue • Neck vein distention • Palpitations • Unexplained weight gain • Dependent edema • Crackles on auscultation	Heart failure
• Hemoptysis • Dyspnea • Wheezing • Chest pain • Fatigue • Weight loss • Fever	Lung and pleural cancer
Pruritus	
• Intense, severe pruritus • Erythematous rash on dry skin at flexion points • Possible edema, scaling, and pustules	Atopic dermatitis
• Scalp excoriation from scratching • Matted, foul-smelling, lusterless hair • Occipital and cervical lymphadenopathy • Oval, gray-white nits on hair shafts	Pediculosis capitis (head lice)
• Gradual or sudden pruritus • Ammonia breath odor • Oliguria or anuria • Fatigue • Irritability • Muscle cramps	Chronic renal failure

(continued)

Integumentary system: Interpreting your findings
(continued)

Sign or symptom and findings	Probable cause
Urticaria	
• Rapid eruption of diffuse urticaria and angioedema, with wheals ranging from pinpoint to palm-size or larger • Pruritic, stinging lesions • Profound anxiety • Weakness • Shortness of breath • Nasal congestion • Dysphagia • Warm, moist skin	Anaphylaxis
• Nonpitting, nonpruritic edema of an extremity or the face • Possibly acute laryngeal edema	Hereditary angioedema
• Erythema chronicum migrans that results in urticaria • Constant malaise and fatigue • Fever • Chills • Lymphadenopathy • Neurologic and cardiac abnormalities • Arthritis	Lyme disease

Common signs and symptoms

A patient may seek care for any of a number of signs and symptoms related to the integumentary system. Some common ones are alopecia, clubbed nails, pruritus, and urticaria. The following history and physical assessment tips will help you assess each one quickly and accurately.

ALOPECIA

Alopecia usually affects the scalp and develops gradually. It can be classified as diffuse or patchy, and scarring or nonscarring. Scarring alopecia, or permanent hair loss, results from hair follicle destruction, which smooths the skin surface, erasing follicular openings. Nonscarring alopecia, or temporary hair loss, results from hair follicle damage that spares follicular openings, allowing future hair growth.

History

If the patient isn't receiving chemotherapeutic drugs or radiation therapy, begin by asking when he first noticed the hair loss or thinning. Does it affect the scalp alone or occur elsewhere on the body? Is it accompanied by itching or rashes? Then carefully explore other signs and symptoms to help distinguish between normal and pathologic hair loss. Ask about recent weight change, anorexia, nausea, vomiting, and altered bowel habits. Also ask about urine changes, such as hematuria or oliguria. Has the patient been especially tired or irritable? Does he have a cough or difficulty breathing? Ask about joint pain or stiffness and about heat or cold intolerance. Inquire about exposure to insecticides.

If the patient is a woman, find out if she has had menstrual irregularities, and note her pregnancy history. If the patient is a man, ask about sexual dysfunction, such as decreased libido or impotence.

Next, ask about hair care. Does the patient frequently use a hot blow dryer or electric curlers? Does he periodically dye, bleach, or perm his hair? Has he changed hair care products lately? Ask a black patient if he uses a hot comb to straighten his hair or a long-toothed comb to achieve an afro look. Does he ever braid the hair in cornrows?

Check for a family history of alopecia, and ask what age relatives were when they started experiencing hair loss. Also ask about nervous habits, such as pulling the hair or twirling it around a finger.

Physical assessment

Begin the physical examination by assessing the extent and pattern of scalp hair loss. Is it patchy or symmetrical? Is the hair surrounding a bald area brit-

tle or lusterless? Is it a different color from other scalp hair? Does it fall out easily? Inspect the underlying skin for follicular openings, erythema, loss of pigment, scaling, induration, broken hair shafts, and hair regrowth.

Then examine the rest of the skin. Note the size, color, texture, and location of any lesions. Check for jaundice, edema, hyperpigmentation, pallor, or duskiness. Examine the patient's nails for vertical or horizontal pitting, thickening, brittleness, or whitening. As you do so, watch for fine tremors in the hands. Observe the patient for muscle weakness and ptosis. Palpate for lymphadenopathy, enlarged thyroid or salivary glands, and masses in the abdomen or chest.

Analysis

One of the most common causes of alopecia is the use of certain chemotherapeutic drugs. Alopecia may also result from the use of other drugs; radiation therapy; a skin, connective tissue, endocrine, nutritional, or psychological disorder; a neoplasm; an infection; a burn; or exposure to toxins.

Normally, everyone loses about 50 hairs per day, and these hairs are replaced by new ones. However, aging, genetic predisposition, and hormonal changes may contribute to gradual hair thinning and hairline recession. This type of alopecia occurs in about 40% of adult men and may also occur in postmenopausal women.

In men, hair loss commonly affects the temporal areas, producing an M-shaped hairline. In women, diffuse thinning marks the centrofrontal area. In both sexes, hair loss also occurs on the trunk, pubic area, axillae, arms, and legs. Another normal pattern of alopecia occurs 2 to 4 months postpartum. This temporary, diffuse hair loss on the scalp may be scant or dramatic and possibly accentuated at the frontal areas. Anxiety, high fever, and even certain hair styles or grooming methods may also cause alopecia.

PEDIATRIC TIP

Alopecia normally occurs during the first 6 months of life, as either a sudden, diffuse hair loss or a gradual thinning that's hardly noticeable. Reassure the infant's parents that this hair loss is normal and temporary. If bald areas result because the infant is left in one position for too long, advise the parents to change his position regularly.

Common causes of alopecia in children include use of chemotherapy or radiation therapy, seborrheic dermatitis (known as cradle cap in infancy), alopecia mucinosa, tinea capitis, and hypopituitarism. Tinea capitis may produce a kerion lesion—a boggy, raised, tender, and hairless lesion. Trichotillomania, a psychological disorder more common in children than adults, may produce patchy baldness with stubby hair growth due to habitual hair pulling. Other causes include progeria and congenital hair shaft defects such as trichorrhexis nodosa.

GERIATRIC TIP

Older patients have thinner hair because of a decrease in hair follicles. Pubic, axillae, and body hair decrease with aging. Balding is more common in men and occurs from the periphery of the scalp and moves to the center. Elderly women may have hair growth on the chin due to hormonal changes.

CLUBBING

A nonspecific sign of pulmonary and cyanotic cardiovascular disorders, clubbing is the painless, usually bilateral increase in soft tissue around the terminal phalanges of the fingers or toes. It doesn't involve changes in the underlying bone. In early clubbing, the normal 160-degree angle between the nail and the nail base approximates 180 degrees. As clubbing progresses, this angle widens and the base of the nail becomes visibly swollen. In late clubbing, the angle where the nail meets the now-convex nail base extends more than halfway up the nail.

History

Because clubbing is usually detected while other symptoms of pulmonary or cardiovascular disease are being evaluated, you should review the patient's current plan of treatment; clubbing may resolve with correction of the underlying disorder.

Physical assessment

Evaluate the extent of clubbing in fingers and toes. Don't mistake curved nails, a normal variation, for clubbing. To quickly examine a patient's fingers for early clubbing, gently palpate the nail bases. Normally, they feel firm, but in early clubbing, nail bases feel springy when palpated. To evaluate late clubbing, have the patient place the first phalanges of the forefingers together, gently pressing the fingernails together. Normal nail bases are concave and create a small, diamond-shaped space when the first phalanges are opposed. In late clubbing, however, the now convex nail bases can touch without leaving a space.

Analysis

Clubbing is typically a sign of pulmonary or cardiovascular disease, such as emphysema, chronic bronchitis, lung cancer, or heart failure. Although clubbing may also result from such hepatic and GI disorders as cirrhosis, Crohn's disease, and ulcerative colitis, it occurs only rarely in these disorders. So first check for more common signs and symptoms.

PEDIATRIC TIP

In children, clubbing is most common in those with cyanotic congenital heart disease and in those with cystic fibrosis. Surgical correction of heart defects may reverse clubbing.

GERIATRIC TIP

Arthritic deformities of the fingers or toes may disguise the presence of clubbing.

PRURITUS

This unpleasant itching sensation usually provokes scratching as the patient tries to gain relief. It affects the skin, certain mucous membranes, and the eyes. Most severe at night, pruritus may be exacerbated by increased skin temperature, poor skin turgor, local vasodilation, dermatoses, and stress.

History

If the patient reports pruritus, ask him when it started and have him describe its onset, frequency, and intensity. If pruritus occurs at night, ask him whether it prevents him from falling asleep or awakens him after he falls asleep. (Generally, pruritus related to dermatoses prevents—but doesn't disturb—sleep.) Is the itching localized or generalized? When is it most severe?

How long does it last? Is there a relationship to such activities as physical exertion, bathing, use of skin care products, or use of colognes or perfume?

Ask the patient how he cleans his skin. In particular, look for excessive bathing, harsh soaps, contact allergy, and excessively hot water. Has he recently changed or added any new skin care products? Does he have occupational exposure to known skin irritants, such as glass fiber insulation or chemicals? Ask about the patient's general health and the medications he takes; new medications are suspect. Has he recently traveled abroad? Does he have pets? Does anyone else in the house report itching? Ask about contact with skin irritants, previous skin disorders, and related symptoms. Then obtain a complete drug history.

Physical assessment

Examine the patient for signs of scratching, such as excoriation, purpura, scabs, scars, or lichenification. Look for primary lesions to help confirm dermatoses.

Analysis

The most common symptom of dermatologic disorders, pruritus may also result from a local or systemic disorder or from use of certain drugs. Physiologic pruritus, such as pruritic urticarial papules and plaques of pregnancy, may occur in primigravidas late in the third trimester. Pruritus can also stem from emotional upset or contact with skin irritants.

PEDIATRIC TIP

Many adult disorders also cause pruritus in children, but they may affect different parts of the body. For instance, scabies may affect the head in infants, but not in adults. Pityriasis rosea may affect the face, hands, and feet of adolescents.

Some childhood diseases, such as measles and chickenpox, can cause pruritus. Hepatic diseases can also produce pruritus in children as bile salts accumulate on the skin.

GERIATRIC TIP
Older patients' skin may feel drier than younger patients' due to decreased sebum production. They are more prone to pruritus from dry skin. Liver and renal disease seen more often in older patients can also cause pruritus.

URTICARIA
Also known as hives, urticaria is a vascular skin reaction characterized by the eruption of transient pruritic wheals—smooth, slightly elevated patches with well-defined erythematous margins and pale centers. It's produced by the local release of histamine or other vasoactive substances as part of a hypersensitivity reaction.

History
If the patient isn't in distress, obtain a complete history. Does the urticaria follow a seasonal pattern? Do certain foods or drugs seem to aggravate it? Is there any relationship to physical exertion? Is the patient routinely exposed to chemicals on the job or at home? Obtain a detailed drug history, including use of prescription and over-the-counter drugs. Note any history of chronic or parasitic infections, skin disease, or GI disorders.

Physical assessment
Fully evaluate the lesions—note their color, configuration, and location on the patient's body.

Analysis
Acute urticaria evolves rapidly and usually has a detectable cause, such as hypersensitivity to a certain drug, food, insect bite, inhalant, or contactant; emotional stress; or an environmental factor. Although individual lesions usually subside within 12 to 24 hours, new crops of lesions may erupt continuously, thus prolonging the attack.

Urticaria lasting longer than 6 weeks is classified as chronic. The lesions may recur for months or years, and the underlying cause is usually unknown. Occasionally, a diagnosis of psychogenic urticaria is made.

Angioedema, or giant urticaria, is characterized by the acute eruption of wheals involving the mucous membranes and, occasionally, the arms, legs, or genitals.

PEDIATRIC TIP
Pediatric forms of urticaria include acute papular urticaria, which usually occurs after an insect bite, and urticaria pigmentosa, which is rare. Hereditary angioedema may be causative.

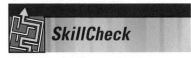

SkillCheck

1. What is the normal angle of the nail base?
   a. 150 degrees
   b. 160 degrees
   c. 170 degrees
   d. 180 degrees

Answer: b. Although values may vary, 160 degrees is the normal angle of the nail base; anything greater suggests clubbing.

2. Which skin lesions glow when transilluminated with a penlight?
   a. Macules
   b. Papules
   c. Hives
   d. Vesicles

Answer: d. Vesicles are fluid-filled lesions that glow when transilluminated.

3. Angioedema is associated with:
   a. urticaria.
   b. pruritus.
   c. hair loss.
   d. clubbing.

Answer: a. Angioedema, also called giant urticaria, is characterized by the acute eruption of wheals involving the mucous membranes and, occasionally, the arms, legs, and genitalia.

4. Asymmetrical borders on a skin lesion suggest:
   a. the lesion is benign.
   b. the lesion is malignant.
   c. nothing in particular; it's a normal variation.
   d. hives have erupted.

Answer: b. An asymmetrical lesion with an irregular border may indicate malignancy.

5. Skin temperature is best assessed with:
   a. the palmar surface of the hands.
   b. the fingers.
   c. the dorsal surfaces of the hands and fingers.
   d. the forearm.

Answer: c. The dorsal surfaces of the hands and fingers are the most sensitive to changes in temperature.

Breasts and axillae

Breast cancer is the most common cancer among women. Increasingly prominent in the news, more women are aware of the disease's risk factors, treatments, and diagnostic measures, and early detection has resulted in increased survival rates. By staying informed and performing breast self-examinations regularly, women can take control of their health and seek medical care when they notice a change in their breasts.

This chapter will help you focus in on common problems related to the breasts and axillae. With a review of anatomy and physiology, physical assessment techniques, and 3-minute assessment guidelines, you'll be ready to evaluate your patient's problems quickly and accurately.

Anatomy and physiology

The breasts, also called mammary glands in women, lie on the anterior chest wall. (See *The female breast.*) They're located vertically between the second or third and the sixth or seventh ribs over the pectoralis major muscle and the serratus anterior muscle, and horizontally between the sternal border and the midaxillary line.

Each breast has a centrally located nipple of pigmented erectile tissue ringed by an areola that's darker than the adjacent tissue. Sebaceous glands, also called Montgomery's tubercles, are scattered on the areola surface, along with hair follicles.

Beneath the skin are glandular, fibrous, and fatty tissues that vary in proportion with age, weight, sex, and other factors such as pregnancy.

A small triangle of tissue, called the tail of Spence, projects into the axilla. Attached to the chest wall musculature are fibrous bands, called Cooper's ligaments, that support each breast.

In women, each breast is surrounded by 12 to 25 glandular lobes containing alveoli that produce milk. The lactiferous ducts from each lobe transport milk to the nipple. In men, the breast has a nipple, an areola, and mostly flat tissue bordering the chest wall.

The breasts also hold several lymph node chains, each serving different areas. (See *Lymph node chains.*) The pectoral lymph nodes drain lymph fluid from most of the breast and anterior chest. The brachial nodes drain most of the arm. The subscapular nodes drain the posterior chest wall and part of the arm. The midaxillary nodes, located near the ribs and the serratus anterior muscle high in the axillae, are the central draining nodes for the pectoral, brachial, and subscapular nodes.

A CLOSER LOOK

The female breast

The illustration below shows a lateral cross section of a woman's breast.

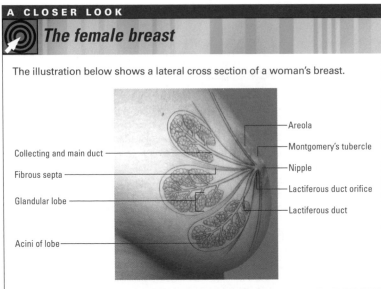

- Areola
- Montgomery's tubercle
- Nipple
- Lactiferous duct orifice
- Lactiferous duct
- Collecting and main duct
- Fibrous septa
- Glandular lobe
- Acini of lobe

A CLOSER LOOK

Lymph node chains

This illustration shows the different lymph node chains in the breast, axilla, and upper arm.

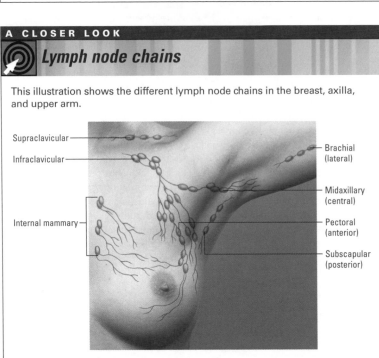

- Supraclavicular
- Infraclavicular
- Internal mammary
- Brachial (lateral)
- Midaxillary (central)
- Pectoral (anterior)
- Subscapular (posterior)

In men and women, the lymphatic system is the most common route of spread of cells that cause breast cancer.

Physical assessment

Having a breast examination can be stressful for a woman. To reduce your patient's anxiety, provide privacy, make her as comfortable as possible, and explain what the examination involves. (See *Breasts and axillae: Normal findings.*)

EXAMINING THE BREASTS

Before examining the breasts, make sure the room is well lighted. Have the patient disrobe from the waist up and sit with her arms at her sides. Keep both breasts uncovered so you can observe them simultaneously to detect differences.

Inspection

Breast skin should be smooth, undimpled, and the same color as the rest of the skin. Check for edema, which can accompany lymphatic obstruction and may signal cancer. Note breast size and symmetry. Asymmetry may occur normally in some adult women, with the left breast usually larger than the right. Inspect the nipples, noting their size and shape. If a nipple is inverted (dimpled or creased), ask the patient when she first noticed the inversion.

Next, inspect the patient's breast while she holds her arms over her head, and then again while she has her hands on her hips. Having the patient assume these positions will help you detect skin or nipple dimpling that might not have been obvious before.

If the patient has large or pendulous breasts, have her stand with her hands on the back of a chair and lean forward. This position helps reveal subtle breast or nipple asymmetry.

If nipple discharge is present and the patient isn't pregnant or breast-feeding, assess the color, consistency, and quantity of the discharge. If possible, obtain a cytologic smear.

Palpation

Before palpating the breasts, ask the patient to lie in a supine position, and place a small pillow under her shoulder on the side you're examining. This causes the breast on that side to protrude. Keep the opposite breast covered for patient's modesty.

Have the patient put her hand on the side you're examining behind her head. This spreads the breast more evenly across the chest and makes finding nodules easier. If her breasts are small, she can leave her arm at her side.

Use your three middle fingers to palpate the breast systematically. Rotating your fingers gently against the chest wall, move in concentric circles. Make sure you include the tail of Spence in your examination.

To perform palpation, place your fingers flat on the breast and compress the tissues gently against the chest wall, palpating in concentric circles outward from the nipple. Palpate the entire breast, including the periphery, tail of Spence, and areola. If the patient has pendulous breasts, palpate down or across the breast with her sitting upright.

As you palpate, note the consistency of the breast tissue. Normal consistency varies widely, depending in part on the proportions of fat and glandular tis-

CHECKLIST
Breasts and axillae: Normal findings

Inspection
❑ Breast skin is smooth, undimpled, and the same color as the rest of the skin.
❑ Breasts are slightly asymmetrical. (The left breast is usually larger than the right.)
❑ No edema, erythema, skin or nipple dimpling, or nipple discharge is apparent.

❑ Nipples are round and protrude.
Palpation
❑ No nodules or unusual tenderness is apparent.
❑ The inframammary ridge at the lower edge of the breast is firm.
❑ Axillary nodes feel soft, small, and nontender.

---

sue and on hormonal influence. Check for nodules and unusual tenderness. Remember that nodularity, fullness, and mild tenderness are premenstrual signs and symptoms. Be sure to ask your patient where she is in her menstrual cycle.

Tenderness may also be related to cysts and cancer. A lump or mass that feels different from the rest of the breast tissue may indicate a pathologic change and warrants further investigation by a physician. If you find what you think is an abnormality, check the other breast, too. Keep in mind that the inframammary ridge at the lower edge of the breast is normally firm and may be mistaken for a tumor.

If you palpate a mass, record the following characteristics:
■ size in centimeters
■ shape (round, discoid, regular, or irregular)
■ consistency (soft, firm, or hard)
■ mobility
■ degree of tenderness
■ location, using the quadrant or clock method. (See *Identifying locations of breast lesions,* page 164.)

To obtain a smear, put on gloves, place a glass slide over the nipple, and smear the discharge on the slide. Spray the slide with a fixative, label it with the patient's name and the date, and send it to the laboratory, according to facility policy.

Be sure to palpate the hollow ductal area beneath the nipple.

EXAMINING THE AXILLAE
To examine the axillae, use inspection and palpation. With the patient sitting or standing, inspect the skin of the axillae for rashes, infections, or unusual pigmentation. Before palpating, ask the patient to relax her arm on the side you're examining. Support her elbow with one of your hands. Cup the fingers of your other hand, and reach high into the apex of the axilla. Place your fingers directly behind the pectoral muscles, pointing toward the midclavicle. (See *Palpating the axillae,* page 165.)

First, try to palpate the central nodes by pressing your fingers downward and in toward the chest wall. You can usually palpate one or more of the nodes, which should be soft, small, and nontender. If you feel a hard, large, or

Identifying locations of breast lesions

Mentally divide the breast into four quadrants and a fifth segment, the tail of Spence. Describe your findings according to the appropriate quadrant or segment. You can also think of the breast as a clock, with the nipple in the center. Then specify locations according to the time (2 o'clock, for example). Either way, specify the location of a lesion or other findings by the distance in centimeters from the nipple.

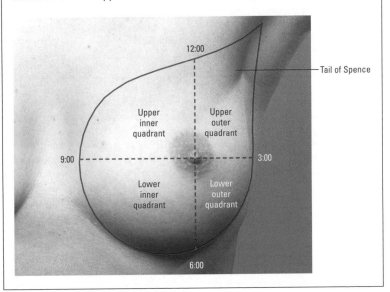

tender lesion, try to palpate the other groups of lymph nodes for comparison.

To palpate the pectoral and anterior nodes, grasp the anterior axillary fold between your thumb and fingers and palpate inside the borders of the pectoral muscles. Palpate the lateral nodes by pressing your fingers along the upper inner arm. Try to compress these nodes against the humerus. To palpate the subscapular or posterior nodes, stand behind the patient and press your fingers to feel the inside of the muscle of the posterior axillary fold.

If the axillary nodes appear abnormal, assess the nodes in the clavicular area. To do this, have the patient relax her neck muscles by flexing her head slightly forward. Stand in front of her, and hook your fingers over the clavicle beside the sternocleidomastoid muscle. Rotate your fingers deeply into this area to feel the supraclavicular nodes.

Palpating the axillae

To palpate the axillae, have the patient sit or lie down. Wear gloves if an ulceration or discharge is present. Ask her to relax her arm, and support it with your nondominant hand.

Keeping the fingers of your dominant hand together, reach high into the apex of the axillae, as shown. Position your fingers so they're directly behind the pectoral muscles, pointing toward the mid-clavicle. Sweep your fingers downward against the ribs and serratus anterior muscle to palpate the midaxillary or central lymph nodes.

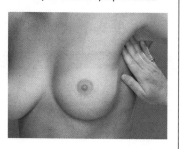

Guidelines for a 3-minute assessment

A 3-minute assessment of signs or symptoms relating to the breasts and axillae includes making general observations, checking the patient's vital signs, and focusing on the patient's chief sign or symptom. However, menses, certain prescription drugs, pregnancy, and other conditions can cause changes in the breast; therefore, you might have trouble differentiating the abnormal from the normal. This section will help you evaluate signs and symptoms rapidly.

MAKING GENERAL OBSERVATIONS

Observe the patient's level of consciousness, chest shape, and condition of the skin over the breasts.

Level of consciousness

Note whether the patient seems anxious or is in pain.

Chest shape

Observe the position, location, and size of the breasts, noting any deviations.

Skin condition

Survey the skin over both breasts. It should be the same color as the rest of the skin. Note obvious lumps or masses, the condition of the nipple, and skin abnormalities, such as dimpling or peau d'orange (orange-peel appearance of an area of skin). Also note skin ulcerations or nipple discharge.

CHECKING VITAL SIGNS

Take your patient's vital signs and compare them with baseline measurements. Check the patient's temperature if you suspect an infection.

FOCUSING ON THE CHIEF SIGN OR SYMPTOM

After you've made general observations and checked the patient's vital signs, you'll want to focus on the patient's chief sign or symptom related to the breasts and axillae for the history and physical assessment.

Further assessment

Although these signs and symptoms don't usually result from problems outside of the breasts and axillae, you may need to assess other body systems to gather additional information.

After you've obtained the necessary information about the patient's reason for seeking care and completed your physical assessment, you'll begin to formulate a diagnostic impression. (See *Breasts and axillae: Interpreting your findings.*)

DIAGNOSTIC IMPRESSION

 Breasts and axillae: Interpreting your findings

After you assess the patient, a group of findings may lead you to suspect a particular disorder. The chart below shows you some common groups of findings for the chief signs and symptoms of the breasts and axillae, along with their probable causes.

Sign or symptom and findings	Probable cause
Breast dimpling	
• Firm, irregular, painful lump • Nipple retraction, deviation, inversion, or flattening • Enlarged axillary lymph nodes	Breast abscess
• History of trauma to fatty tissue of the breast (patient may not remember such trauma) • Tenderness and erythema • Bruising • Hard, indurated, poorly delineated lump that's fibrotic and fixed to underlying tissue or overlying skin • Signs of nipple retraction	Fat necrosis
• Heat • Erythema • Swelling • Pain and tenderness • Flulike signs and symptoms, such as fever, malaise, fatigue, and aching	Mastitis

Breasts and axillae: Interpreting your findings (continued)

Sign or symptom and findings	Probable cause
Breast nodule	
• Single nodule that feels firm, elastic, and round or lobular, with well-defined margins • Extremely mobile, "slippery" feel • No pain or tenderness • Size varies from that of a pinhead to very large • Grows rapidly • Usually located around the nipple or on the lateral side of the upper outer quadrant	Adenofibroma
• Unilateral with irregular, poorly delineated borders • Usually hard, nontender, and fixed to the underlying tissue • Breast dimpling • Nipple deviation or retraction • Almost one-half are located in the upper outer quadrant • Nontender • Serous or bloody discharge • Edema or peau d'orange of the skin overlying the mass • Axillary lymphadenopathy	Breast cancer
• Smooth, round, slightly elastic nodules • Increase in size and tenderness just before menstruation • Mobile • Clear, watery (serous), or sticky nipple discharge • Bloating • Irritability • Abdominal cramping	Fibrocystic breast disease
Breast pain	
• Tender, palpable abscesses on the periphery of the areola • Fever • Inflamed sebaceous Montgomery's glands	Areolar gland abscess
• Unilateral breast pain or tenderness • Serous or bloody nipple discharge, usually only from one duct • Small, soft, poorly delineated mass in the ducts beneath the areola	Intraductal papilloma

(continued)

Breasts and axillae: Interpreting your findings *(continued)*

Sign or symptom and findings	Probable cause
Breast pain *(continued)*	
• Small, well-delineated nodule • Localized erythema • Induration	Sebaceous cyst (infected)
Nipple retraction	
• Poorly defined, rubbery nodule beneath the areola with a blue-green discoloration • Areolar burning, itching, swelling, tenderness, and erythema • Nipple pain with a thick, sticky, grayish, multiductal discharge	Mammary duct ectasia
• History of breast surgery that may have caused underlying scarring	Surgery

Common signs and symptoms

A patient may seek care for any of a number of signs and symptoms related to the breasts and axillae. Some common ones are breast dimpling, breast nodules, breast pain, and nipple retraction.

BREAST DIMPLING

Breast dimpling is the puckering or retraction of skin on the breast. Dimpling usually affects women older than age 40 but also occasionally occurs in men.

History

Obtain a medical, reproductive, and family history, noting factors that place the patient at high risk for breast cancer. Ask about pregnancy history because women who haven't had a full-term pregnancy until after age 30 are at higher risk for developing breast cancer. Has her mother or a sister had breast cancer? Has she herself had a previous malignancy, especially cancer in the other breast? Ask about the patient's dietary habits because a high-fat diet predisposes women to breast cancer.

Ask the patient if she has noticed changes in the shape of the breast. Is any area painful or tender, and is the pain cyclic? If she's breast-feeding, has she recently experienced high temperature, chills, malaise, muscle aches, fatigue, or other flulike signs or symptoms? Can she remember sustaining any trauma to the breast?

Physical assessment

Carefully inspect the dimpled area. Is it swollen, red, or warm to the touch? Do you see bruises or contusions? Ask the patient to tense her pectoral muscles by pressing down on her hips with both hands or by raising her hands over her head. Does puckering increase? Gently pull the skin upward toward the clavicle. Is dimpling exaggerated?

Observe the breast for nipple retraction. Do both nipples point in the same direction? Are the nipples flattened or inverted? Does the patient report nipple discharge? If so, ask her to describe the color and character of the discharge. Observe the contour of both breasts. Are they symmetrical?

Examine both breasts with your patient in supine, sitting, and forward-leaning positions. Does the skin move freely over both breasts? If you can palpate a lump, describe its size, location, consistency, mobility, and delineation. What relation does the lump have to breast dimpling? Gently mold the breast skin around the lump. Is dimpling exaggerated? Also, examine breast and axillary lymph nodes, noting any enlargement.

Analysis

Breast dimpling results from abnormal attachment of the skin to underlying tissue. It suggests an inflammatory or malignant mass beneath the skin surface and usually represents a late sign of breast cancer; benign lesions usually don't produce this effect.

Because breast dimpling occurs over a mass or induration, the patient usually discovers other signs before becoming aware of this one. However, a thorough breast examination may reveal dimpling and alert the patient and nurse to a problem.

PEDIATRIC TIP

Because breast cancer, the most likely cause of dimpling, is extremely rare in children, consider trauma a likely cause. As in adults, breast dimpling may occur in adolescents from fatty tissue necrosis caused by trauma.

BREAST NODULES

A breast nodule, or lump, may be found in any part of the breast, including in the axilla.

History

If your patient reports a lump, ask how and when she discovered it.

Does the size and tenderness of the lump vary with her menstrual cycle? Has the lump changed since she first noticed it? Has she noticed other breast signs, such as a change in breast shape, size, or contour; a discharge; or a change in the nipples?

Is she breast-feeding? Does she have fever, chills, fatigue, or other flulike signs and symptoms? Ask her to describe any pain or tenderness associated with the lump. Is the pain in one breast only? Has she sustained recent trauma to the breast?

Explore the patient's medical and family history for factors that increase her risk of breast cancer. These include following a high-fat diet, having a mother or sister with breast cancer, or having a history of cancer, especially in the other breast. Other risk factors include nulliparity and a first pregnancy after age 30.

Physical assessment

Perform a thorough breast examination. Pay special attention to the upper outer quadrant of each breast, where half the ductal tissue is located. This is the most common site of malignant breast tumors.

Carefully palpate a suspected breast nodule, noting its location, shape, size, consistency, mobility, and delineation. Does the nodule feel soft, rubbery, and elastic or hard? Is it mobile, slipping away from your fingers as you palpate it, or firmly fixed to the adjacent tissue? Does the nodule seem to limit the mobility of the entire breast? Note the nodule's delineation. Are the borders clearly defined or indefinite? Or does the area feel more like a hardness or diffuse induration than a nodule with definite borders?

Do you feel one nodule or several small ones? Is the shape round, oval, lobular, or irregular? Inspect and palpate the skin over the nodule for warmth, redness, and edema. Palpate the lymph nodes of the breast and axilla for enlargement.

Observe the contour of the breasts, looking for asymmetry and irregularities. Be alert for signs of retraction, such as skin dimpling and nipple deviation, retraction, or flattening. (To exaggerate dimpling, have your patient raise her arms over her head or press her hands against her hips.) Gently pull the breast skin toward the clavicle. Is dimpling evident? Mold the breast tissue and again observe for dimpling.

Be alert for a nipple discharge that's spontaneous, unilateral, and nonmilky (serous, bloody, or purulent). Be careful not to confuse it with the grayish discharge that can often be elicited from the nipples of a woman who has been pregnant.

Analysis

A breast nodule is a commonly reported gynecologic sign that has two chief causes: benign breast disease and cancer. Benign breast disease, the leading cause of nodules, can stem from cyst formation in obstructed and dilated lactiferous ducts, hypertrophy or tumor formation in the ductal system, and inflammation or infection.

Although fewer than 20% of breast nodules are malignant, the signs of breast cancer aren't easily distinguished from those of benign breast disease. Breast cancer is a leading cause of death among women but can occur occasionally in men, with signs and symptoms mimicking those found in women. Thus, breast nodules in both sexes should always be evaluated.

A woman who's familiar with the feel of her breasts and performs monthly breast self-examination can detect a nodule that's less than 5 mm in size—considerably smaller than the 1-cm nodule that's readily detectable by an experienced examiner. However, a woman may fail to report a nodule for fear of breast cancer.

PEDIATRIC TIP

Most nodules in children and adolescents reflect the normal response of breast tissue to hormonal fluctuations. For instance, the breasts of young teenage girls may normally contain cordlike nodules that become tender just before menstruation.

A transient breast nodule in young boys (as well as women between ages 20 and 30) may result from juvenile mastitis, which usually affects one breast. Signs of inflammation are present in a firm mass beneath the nipple.

In women age 70 and older, 75% of all breast lumps are malignant.

BREAST PAIN

An unreliable indicator of cancer, breast pain (also known as mastalgia) commonly results from benign breast disease. It may occur during rest or movement and may be aggravated by manipulation or palpation. (Breast tenderness refers to pain elicited by physical contact.) Breast pain may be unilateral or bilateral; cyclic, intermittent, or constant; and dull or sharp.

History

Begin by asking the patient if breast pain is constant or intermittent. For either type, ask about onset and character. If intermittent, determine the relationship of pain to the phase of the menstrual cycle. Is the patient breast-feeding? If not, ask about nipple discharge, and have her describe it. Is she pregnant? Has she reached menopause? Has she recently experienced flulike symptoms or sustained an injury to the breast? Has she noticed change in breast shape or contour?

Ask your patient to describe the pain. She may describe it as sticking, stinging, shooting, stabbing, throbbing, or burning. Determine if the pain affects one breast or both, and ask the patient to point to the painful area.

Physical assessment

Instruct the patient to place her arms at her sides, and inspect her breasts. Note their size, symmetry, and contour and the appearance of the skin. Remember that breast shape and size vary widely and that breasts normally change during the menstrual cycle, pregnancy, breast-feeding, and aging. Are the breasts red or edematous? Are the veins prominent?

Note the size, shape, and symmetry of the nipples and areolae. Do you detect ecchymosis, a rash, ulceration, or a discharge? Do the nipples point in the same direction? Do you see signs of retraction, such as skin dimpling or nipple inversion or flattening? Repeat your inspection, first with the patient's arms raised above her head and then with her hands pressed against her hips.

Palpate the patient's breasts, first with her seated and then with her lying down and a pillow placed under her shoulder on the side being examined. Use the pads of your fingers to compress breast tissue against the chest wall. Proceed systematically from the sternum to the midline and from the axilla to the midline, noting warmth, tenderness, nodules, masses, or irregularities. Palpate the nipple, noting tenderness and nodules, and check for discharge. Palpate axillary lymph nodes, noting any enlargement.

Analysis

Breast pain may result from surface cuts, furuncles, contusions, and similar lesions (superficial pain); nipple fissures and inflammation in the papillary ducts and areolae (severe, localized pain); stromal distention in the breast parenchyma (tenderness); a tumor that affects nerve endings (severe, constant pain); or inflammatory lesions that not only distend the stroma but also irritate sensory nerve endings (severe, constant pain). Breast pain may radiate to the back, the arms, and sometimes the neck.

Breast tenderness in women may occur before menstruation and during pregnancy. Before menstruation, breast pain or tenderness stems from increased mammary blood flow due to hormonal changes. During pregnancy, breast tenderness and throbbing, tingling, or pricking sensations may occur, also from hormonal changes. In men, breast pain may stem from gynecomastia (especially during puberty and senescence), reproductive tract anomalies, and organic disease of the liver or of the pituitary, adrenal cortex, and thyroid glands.

PEDIATRIC TIP
Transient gynecomastia can cause breast pain in males during puberty.

GERIATRIC TIP
Breast pain secondary to benign breast disease is rare in postmenopausal women. Breast pain can also be caused by trauma from falls or physical abuse. Because of decreased pain perception and decreased cognitive function, elderly patients may fail to report breast pain.

NIPPLE RETRACTION
Nipple retraction, the inward displacement of the nipple below the level of surrounding breast tissue, may indicate an inflammatory breast lesion or cancer.

History
Ask the patient when she first noticed that the nipple was retracted. Has she experienced other nipple changes, such as itching, discoloration, discharge, or excoriation? Has she noticed breast pain, lumps, redness, swelling, or warmth? Obtain a history, noting risk factors of breast cancer, such as a family history or previous malignancy.

Physical assessment
Carefully examine both nipples and breasts with the patient sitting upright with her arms at her sides, with her hands pressing on her hips, and with her arms overhead; and with the patient leaning forward so her breasts hang. Look for redness, excoriation, and discharge; nipple flattening and deviation; and breast asymmetry, dimpling, or contour differences.

Nipple retraction is typically confused with nipple inversion, a common abnormality that's congenital in some patients and doesn't usually signal underlying disease. A retracted nipple appears flat and broad, whereas an inverted nipple can be pulled out from the sulcus where it hides.

Try to evert the nipple by gently squeezing the areola. With the patient in a supine position, palpate both breasts for lumps, especially beneath the areola. Mold breast skin over the lump or gently pull it up toward the clavicle, looking for accentuated nipple retraction. Also, palpate axillary lymph nodes.

Analysis
Nipple retraction results from scar tissue formation within a lesion or large mammary duct. As the scar tissue shortens, it pulls adjacent tissue inward, causing nipple deviation, flattening, and finally retraction.

PEDIATRIC TIP
Nipple retraction doesn't occur in prepubescent females.

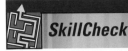
SkillCheck

1. Who can detect the smallest lesions in the breast?
   a. An experienced examiner
   b. A woman who performs breast self-examination every month
   c. A woman who performs breast self-examination twice per year
   d. The woman's physician

Answer: b. The woman who's familiar with the feel of her breasts and performs a breast self-examination every month can detect smaller lesions than an experienced examiner.

2. Breast dimpling usually represents:
   a. a normal finding.
   b. a benign breast lesion.
   c. an early sign of breast cancer.
   d. a late sign of breast cancer.

Answer: d. Breast dimpling usually suggests an inflammatory or malignant mass beneath the skin surface and represents a late sign of breast cancer. Benign lesions usually don't produce this effect.

3. Where is the most common site of malignant breast tumors?
   a. Upper outer quadrant
   b. Upper inner quadrant
   c. Lower inner quadrant
   d. Lower outer quadrant

Answer: a. The upper outer quadrant, where half the ductal tissue is located, is the most common site of malignant breast tumors.

4. Normal premenstrual signs and symptoms include:
   a. nipple discharge and breast tenderness.
   b. breast fullness and mild tenderness.
   c. a single, hard nodule and breast pain.
   d. breast dimpling and peau d'orange.

Answer: b. Keep in mind that normal premenstrual signs and symptoms include breast fullness, mild tenderness, and nodularity. If you find what you think is an abnormality, check the other breast too.

5. Where is the tail of Spence located?
   a. Upper outer quadrant
   b. Upper inner quadrant
   c. Lower inner quadrant
   d. Lower outer quadrant

Answer: a. The tail of Spence is a small triangle of tissue located in the upper outer quadrant.

Female genitourinary system

Disorders of the female genitourinary (GU) system can have wide-ranging effects on other body systems. For example, ovarian dysfunction can alter endocrine balance, and kidney dysfunction can affect the production of the hormone erythropoietin, which regulates red blood cell production.

Assessing the female GU system quickly can be challenging. This chapter can help with a review of anatomy and physiology, essential physical assessment techniques, and 3-minute assessment guidelines for common signs and symptoms of the female GU system.

Anatomy and physiology

The female GU system encompasses the urinary system and reproductive organs and structures.

URINARY SYSTEM

The urinary system consists of the kidneys, ureters, bladder, and urethra. (See *Urinary system.*)

Kidneys

The essential functions of the urinary system—such as forming urine and maintaining homeostasis—take place in the highly vascular kidneys. These bean-shaped organs are $4\frac{1}{2}''$ to $5''$ (11.5 to 12.5 cm) long and $2\frac{1}{2}''$ (6.4 cm) wide. Located retroperitoneally on either side of the lumbar vertebrae, the kidneys lie behind the abdominal organs and in front of the muscles attached to the vertebral column. The peritoneal fat layer protects them.

Crowded by the liver, the right kidney extends slightly lower than the left. Each kidney contains roughly 1 million nephrons. Urine gathers in collecting tubules and ducts and eventually drains into the ureters, down into the bladder and, when urination occurs, out through the urethra.

Ureters

The ureters are $10''$ to $12''$ (25.5 to 30.5 cm) long. The left ureter is slightly longer than the right because of the left kidney's higher position. The diameter of each ureter varies from $\frac{1}{8}''$ to $\frac{1}{4}''$ (0.3 to 0.6 cm), with the narrowest part at the ureteropelvic junction.

Located along the posterior abdominal wall, the ureters enter the bladder anteromedially. They carry urine from the kidneys to the bladder by peristaltic contractions that occur one to five times per minute.

Bladder

Located in the pelvis, the bladder is where urine collects. Bladder capacity

Urinary system

The illustration below shows the main structures of the urinary system.

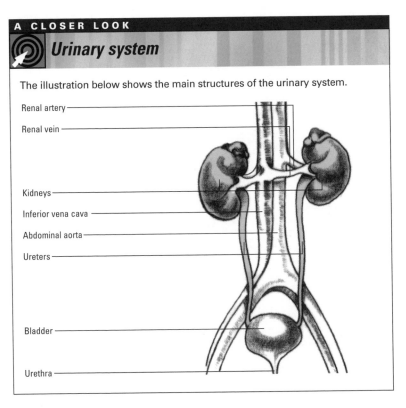

Renal artery
Renal vein
Kidneys
Inferior vena cava
Abdominal aorta
Ureters
Bladder
Urethra

ranges from 500 to 1,000 ml in healthy adults. The bladders of children and elderly patients have a lower capacity. When the bladder is empty, it lies behind the pelvic bone; when it's full, it becomes displaced under the peritoneal cavity.

Urethra

The urethra is a small duct that carries urine from the bladder to the outside of the body. A woman's urethra is only 1″ to 2″ (2.5 to 5 cm) long and opens anterior to the vaginal opening.

REPRODUCTIVE SYSTEM

The female reproductive system consists of external and internal genitalia.

External genitalia

The external genitalia, collectively called the vulva, consist of the mons pubis, labia majora, labia minora, clitoris, vagina, urethra, and Skene's and Bartholin's glands. (See *External genitalia,* page 176.)

The mons pubis is a mound of adipose tissue overlying the symphysis pubis and is covered with pubic hair in the adult. Pubic hair typically appears at age 10½. It may become sparse after menopause due to hormonal changes.

A CLOSER LOOK

External genitalia

The illustration below shows the main parts of the external female genitalia.

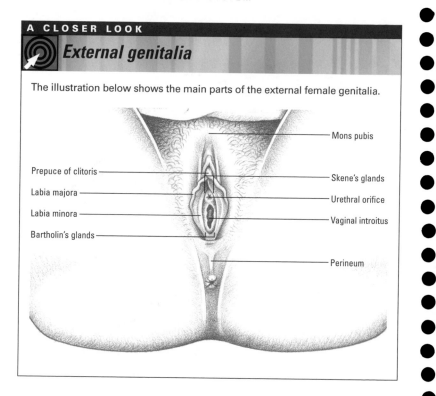

Native Americans and Asians usually have less pubic hair than people of other races.

The outer vulval lips, or labia majora, are two rounded folds of adipose tissue that extend from the mons pubis to the perineum. The labia majora is covered with hair.

The inner vulval lips are called the labia minora. The anterolateral and medial parts join to form the prepuce and frenulum, the folds of skin that cap the clitoris. The posterior union of the labia minora is called the fourchette.

The clitoris is made up of erectile tissue and lies between the labia minora at the top of the vestibule, which contains the urethral and vaginal open-

ings. The urethral opening is a slit below the clitoris.

The vaginal opening, or introitus, is posterior to the urethral orifice. This opening is a thin vertical slit in women with intact hymens and a large opening with irregular edges in women whose hymens have been perforated. In some women, the hymen is absent.

The perineum is the area bordered anteriorly by the top of the labial fold and posteriorly by the anus.

Two kinds of glands have ducts that open into the vulva. Skene's glands are tiny structures just below the urethra, each containing 6 to 31 ducts. Bartholin's glands are found posterior to the vaginal opening. Neither of these

Internal genitalia

The illustration below shows the main internal structures of the female reproductive system.

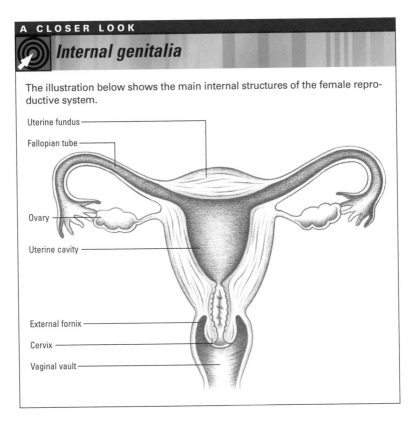

Uterine fundus

Fallopian tube

Ovary

Uterine cavity

External fornix

Cervix

Vaginal vault

---

glands can be seen, but they can be palpated if enlarged.

Skene's and Bartholin's glands produce fluids important for the reproductive process. They can become infected, usually with organisms known to cause sexually transmitted diseases (STDs).

Internal genitalia

The internal genitalia include the vagina, uterus, ovaries, and fallopian tubes. (See *Internal genitalia*.)

A pink, hollow, collapsed tube, the vagina is located between the urethra and the rectum, extending up and back

from the vulva to the uterus. It's the route of passage for childbirth and menses.

The uterus is a hollow, pear-shaped, muscular organ that lies between the rectum and the bladder. It's divided into the fundus and the cervix, which protrudes into the vagina. The cervix contains mucus-secreting glands that help in reproduction and protect the uterus from pathogens. The function of the uterus is to nurture and then expel the fetus.

The position of the uterus in the pelvic cavity may vary, depending on bladder fullness. The uterus may also tip in different directions.

A pair of oval organs about $1^1/_4''$ (3 cm) long, the ovaries are usually found near the lateral pelvic wall at the height of the anterosuperior iliac spine. They produce ova and release the hormones estrogen and progesterone. The ovaries become fully developed after puberty and shrink after menopause.

Each about $4''$ (10 cm) long, the two fallopian tubes extend from the ovaries into the upper portion of the uterus. Their funnel-shaped ends curve toward the ovaries and, during ovulation, help guide the ova to the uterus after expulsion from the ovaries. The fallopian tube is also the usual site of fertilization of the ova by the sperm.

Physical assessment

To perform a physical assessment of the female GU system, you'll use inspection, percussion, and palpation to evaluate the urinary and reproductive systems. (See *Female GU system: Normal findings.*)

EXAMINING THE URINARY SYSTEM
Explain the procedure to the patient, especially before percussing the kidneys. Otherwise, you may startle the patient and mistake her reaction for a feeling of acute tenderness.

Inspection
First, observe the color and shape of the area around the kidneys and bladder. The skin should be free from lesions, discoloration, and swelling.

Percussion
Kidney percussion checks for costovertebral angle tenderness that occurs with inflammation. To percuss over the kidneys, have the patient sit up. Place the ball of your nondominant hand on her back at the costovertebral angle of the 12th rib. Strike the ball of that hand with the ulnar surface of your other hand. Use just enough force to cause a painless but perceptible thud.

To percuss the bladder, first ask the patient to empty it. Then have her lie in the supine position. Start at the symphysis pubis and percuss upward toward the bladder and over it. You should hear tympany. A dull sound signals retained urine.

Palpation
Because the kidneys lie behind other organs and are protected by muscle, they normally aren't palpable unless they're enlarged. However, in very thin patients, you may be able to feel the lower end of the right kidney as a smooth round mass that drops on inspiration.

In elderly patients, you may be able to palpate both kidneys because of decreased muscle tone and elasticity. If the kidneys feel enlarged, the patient may have hydronephrosis, cysts, or tumors.

To palpate the kidneys, first have the patient lie in a supine position. To palpate the right kidney, stand on her right side. Place your left hand under her back and your right hand on her abdomen.

Instruct her to inhale deeply so her kidney moves downward. As she inhales, press up with your left hand and down with your right. Remember, the

Female GU system: Normal findings

Inspection
❑ No lesions, discoloration, or swelling on the skin over the kidneys and bladder areas is apparent.
❑ No discharge or ulcerations from the urethra are apparent.
❑ Labia majora is moist and free from lesions.
❑ Vaginal discharge is normal. (Discharge varies from clear and stretchy to white and opaque, depending on the menstrual cycle; odorless; and nonirritating to the mucosa.)
❑ Cervix looks smooth and round.

Percussion
❑ No costovertebral angle tenderness is apparent.

❑ Tympany is heard over the empty bladder.

Palpation
❑ Kidneys are unpalpable, except in very thin and elderly patients.
❑ Bladder is unpalpable.
❑ Labia feels soft, without swelling, hardness, or tenderness.
❑ Bartholin's glands are unpalpable.
❑ Vaginal wall has no nodularity, tenderness, or bulging.
❑ Cervix is smooth and firm, protrudes ¼″ to 1¼″ (0.5 to 3 cm) into the vagina, and is freely moveable in all directions.

---

kidneys normally aren't palpable unless they're enlarged.

You won't be able to palpate the bladder unless it's distended. With the patient in a supine position, use the fingers of one hand to palpate the lower abdomen in a light dipping motion. A distended bladder will feel firm and relatively smooth. If the patient is 12 weeks or more pregnant, you might actually be feeling the fundus of the uterus, palpable just above the symphysis pubis.

EXAMINING THE REPRODUCTIVE SYSTEM
Before the examination, ask the patient to void, to prevent discomfort and inaccurate findings during palpation. Have her disrobe and put on an examination gown. Help her into the dorsal lithotomy position, and drape all areas not being examined. Make sure you explain the procedure to her.

You'll begin by examining external genitalia and then internal genitalia.

Inspecting the external genitalia
First, put on a pair of gloves. Spread the labia and locate the urethral meatus. It should be a pink, irregular, slit-like opening at the midline, just above the vagina. Note the presence of discharge (a sign of urethral infection) or ulcerations (a sign of an STD).

Inspect the external genitalia and pubic hair to assess sexual maturity. Pubic hair changes in density, color, and texture throughout a woman's life. Before adolescence, the pubic area is covered only with body hair. In adolescence, this hair grows thicker, darker, coarser, and curlier. In full maturity, it spreads over the symphysis pubis and inner thighs. In later years, the hair grows thin, gray, and brittle.

Using your index finger and thumb, gently spread the labia majora and minora. They should be moist and free from lesions. You may detect a normal discharge varying from clear and stretchy before ovulation to white and opaque after ovulation. The discharge should be odorless and nonirritating to the mucosa.

Examine the vestibule, especially the area around the Bartholin's and Skene's glands. Check for swelling, redness, lesions, discharge, and unusual odor. If you detect any of these conditions, notify the physician, and obtain a specimen for culture. Finally, inspect the vaginal opening, noting whether the hymen is intact or perforated.

Palpating the external genitalia

Spread the labia with one hand and palpate with the other. The labia should feel soft. Note swelling, hardness, or tenderness. If you detect a mass or lesion, palpate it to determine its size, shape, and consistency.

If you find swelling or tenderness, see if you can palpate Bartholin's glands, which normally aren't palpable. To do this, insert your finger carefully into the patient's posterior introitus, and place your thumb along the lateral edge of the swollen or tender labium. Gently squeeze the labium. If discharge from the duct results, culture it.

INFLAMED URETHRA

If the urethra is inflamed, milk it and the area of Skene's glands. First, moisten your gloved index finger with water. Then separate the labia with your other hand, and insert your index finger about 1¼″ (3 cm) into the anterior vagina. With the pad of your finger, gently press and pull outward. Continue palpating down to the introitus. This procedure shouldn't cause the patient discomfort. Culture the discharge.

Inspecting the internal genitalia

Nurses don't routinely inspect internal genitalia unless they're in advanced practice. However, you may be asked to assist with this examination. To start, select an appropriate speculum for your patient. A Graves' speculum is usually used. However, if the patient has an intact hymen, has never given birth through the vaginal canal, or has a contracted introitus from menopause, use a Pederson speculum.

Hold the speculum under warm, running water to lubricate and warm the blades. Don't use lubricants; many of them are bacteriostatic and can alter Papanicolaou (Pap) test results.

Sit or stand at the foot of the examination table. Tell the patient she'll feel internal pressure and possibly some slight, transient discomfort as you insert and open the speculum.

Using your dominant hand, hold the speculum by the base with the blades anchored between your index and middle fingers. This keeps the blades from accidentally opening during insertion. Encourage the patient to take slow, deep breaths during insertion to relax her abdominal muscles. (See *Inserting a speculum.*)

After inserting the speculum, observe the color, texture, and integrity of the vaginal lining. A thin, white, odorless discharge on the vaginal walls is normal. Using the thumb of the hand holding the speculum, press the lower lever to open the blades. Lock them in

Inserting a speculum

Proper positioning and insertion of the speculum are important for the patient's comfort and for proper visualization of internal structures. The illustration shows the proper angle and hand position for insertion.

Initial insertion
Place the index and middle fingers of your nondominant hand about 1" (2.5 cm) into the vagina and spread the fingers to exert pressure on the posterior vagina. Hold the speculum in your dominant hand, and insert the blades between your fingers as shown.

Deeper insertion
Ask the patient to bear down to open the introitus and relax the perineal muscles. Point the speculum slightly downward, and insert the blades until the base of the speculum touches your fingers, inside the vagina.

Rotation and opening
Rotate the speculum in the same plane as the vagina, and withdraw your fingers. Open the blades as far as possible and lock them. You should now have a clear view of the cervix.

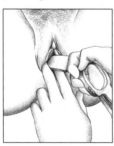 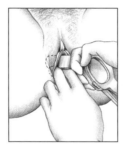 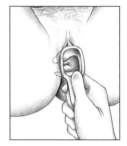

the open position by tightening the thumb screw above the lever.

Examine the cervix for color, position, size, shape, mucosal integrity, and discharge. It should be smooth and round. The central cervical opening, or cervical os, is circular in a woman who hasn't given birth vaginally and a horizontal slit in a woman who has. Expect to see a clear, watery cervical discharge during ovulation and a slightly bloody discharge just before menstruation.

Use the speculum to obtain a specimen for a Pap test. Finally, unlock and close the blades and withdraw the speculum.

Palpating the internal genitalia

To palpate the internal genitalia, lubricate the index and middle fingers of your gloved dominant hand. Stand at the foot of the examination table and position the hand for insertion into the vagina by extending your thumb, index, and middle fingers and curling your ring and little finger toward your palm.

Use the thumb and index finger of your other hand to spread the labia ma-

Performing a bimanual examination

During a bimanual examination, you palpate the uterus and ovaries from the inside and the outside simultaneously. The illustrations below show how to perform such an examination.

1. Assume the proper position

After putting on gloves, place the index and third fingers of your dominant hand in the patient's vagina, and move them up to the cervix. Place the fingers of your other hand on the patient's abdomen between the umbilicus and the symphysis pubis, as shown.

Elevate the cervix and uterus by pressing upward with the two fingers inside the vagina. At the same time, press down and in with the hand on the abdomen. Try to grasp the uterus between your hands.

2. Note the position

Now move your fingers into the posterior fornix, pressing upward and forward to bring the anterior uterine wall up to your nondominant hand. Use your dominant hand to palpate the lower portion of the uterine wall. Note the position of the uterus.

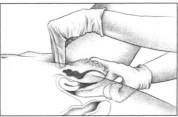

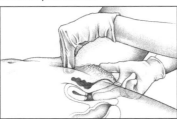

jora. Insert your two lubricated fingers into the vagina, exerting pressure posteriorly to avoid irritating the anterior wall and urethra.

When your fingers are fully inserted, note tenderness or nodularity in the vaginal wall. Ask the patient to bear down so you can assess the support of the vaginal outlet. Bulging of the vaginal wall may indicate a cystocele or rectocele.

To palpate the cervix, sweep your fingers from side to side across the cervix and around the os. The cervix should be smooth and firm and pro-

trude ¼″ to 1¼″ (1.5 to 3.5 cm) into the vagina. If you palpate nodules or irregularities, the patient may have cysts, tumors, or other lesions.

Next, place your fingers into the recessed area around the cervix. The cervix should move in all directions. If the patient reports pain during this part of the examination, she may have inflammation of the uterus or adnexa (ovaries, fallopian tubes, and ligaments of the uterus).

A bimanual examination allows you to palpate the uterus and ovaries. Usually, only nurses in advanced practice

3. Palpate the walls

Slide your fingers farther into the anterior section of the fornix, the space between the uterus and cervix. You should feel part of the posterior uterine wall with this hand. You should feel part of the anterior uterine wall with the fingertips of your nondominant hand. Note the size, shape, surface characteristics, consistency, and mobility of the uterus as well as tenderness.

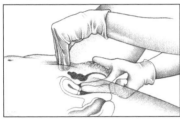

4. Palpate the ovaries

After palpating the anterior and posterior walls of the uterus, move your nondominant hand toward the abdomen's right lower quadrant. Slip the fingers of your dominant hand into the right fornix and palpate the right ovary. Then palpate the left ovary. Note the size, shape, and contour of each ovary. They should be unpalpable in postmenopausal women. Remove your hand from the patient's abdomen and your fingers from her vagina, and discard your gloves.

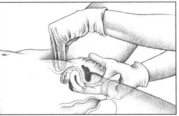

perform bimanual palpation. (See *Performing a bimanual examination.*)

Rectovaginal palpation, the last step in a genital assessment, examines the posterior part of the uterus and pelvic cavity. Warn the patient that this procedure may be uncomfortable.

Put on a new pair of gloves, and apply water-soluble lubricant to the index and middle fingers of your gloved dominant hand. Instruct the patient to bear down with her vaginal and rectal muscles; then insert your index finger a short way into the vagina and your middle finger into the rectum.

Use your middle finger to assess rectal muscle and sphincter tone. Insert your finger deeper into the rectum, and palpate the rectal wall with your middle finger. Sweep the rectum with your fingers, assessing for masses or nodules.

Palpate the posterior wall of the uterus through the anterior wall of the rectum, evaluating the uterus for size, shape, tenderness, and masses. The rectovaginal septum, the wall between the rectum and the vagina, should feel smooth and springy.

Place your nondominant hand on the patient's abdomen at the symphysis pubis. With your index finger in the vagina, palpate deeply to feel the posterior edge of the cervix and the lower posterior wall of the uterus.

When you're finished, discard the gloves and wash your hands. Help the patient to a sitting position, and provide privacy for dressing and personal hygiene.

Guidelines for a 3-minute assessment

If your patient reports having a problem that involves the urinary or reproductive system, you should proceed with a 3-minute assessment. Begin by making some general observations and taking the patient's vital signs. These observations can provide clues about renal dysfunction. Then shift your focus to the patient's chief sign or symptom.

MAKING GENERAL OBSERVATIONS

Your general observations of the patient include checking level of consciousness (LOC) and overall appearance.

Level of consciousness

Observing the patient's behavior can give you clues about her LOC. Does she have trouble concentrating, have memory loss, or seem disoriented? Kidney dysfunction can cause these symptoms. Progressive, chronic kidney failure can cause lethargy, confusion, disorientation, stupor, convulsions, and coma.

Overall appearance

Observe your patient's overall appearance. Note the patient's facial expression for signs of anxiety or pain.

CHECKING VITAL SIGNS

The patient's vital signs and weight can offer important information. For example, a patient's vital signs might reveal hypertension, which can cause renal dysfunction if it's uncontrolled. Check blood pressure in each arm. Take her temperature, noting fever and accompanying chills. Weighing the patient can provide information about fluid status and is important for patients with urinary disorders or renal failure, especially those receiving dialysis. Evaluate for the presence of pain. Obtaining details related to pain, such as quality, intensity, location, and triggering factors, may be helpful in interpreting your findings.

FOCUSING ON THE CHIEF SIGN OR SYMPTOM

After you've made general observations and checked the patient's vital signs, you'll want to focus on the patient's chief GU sign or symptom for the history and physical assessment.

Further assessment

Assessment of other body systems, such as the GI and neurologic systems, may provide additional information.

After obtaining a history and performing a physical assessment, you'll begin to form a diagnostic impression. (See *Female GU system: Interpreting your findings,* pages 186 to 188.)

Common signs and symptoms

A woman may seek care for any number of signs and symptoms related to the GU system. Some common ones are dysmenorrhea, dysuria, urinary incontinence, and vaginal discharge.

DYSMENORRHEA

Dysmenorrhea—painful menstruation—affects over 50% of menstruating women; in fact, it's the leading cause of lost time from school and work among women of childbearing age. Dysmenorrhea may involve sharp, intermittent pain or dull, aching pain. It's usually characterized by mild to severe cramping or colicky pain in the pelvis or lower abdomen that may radiate to the thighs and lower sacrum. This pain may precede menses by several days or may accompany it. The pain gradually subsides as bleeding tapers off.

History

If the patient complains of dysmenorrhea, have her describe it fully. Is it in-termittent or continuous? Sharp, cramping, or aching? Ask where the pain is located and whether it's bilateral. How long has she been experiencing it? When does the pain begin and end, and when is it severe? Does it radiate to the back? Explore associated signs and symptoms, such as nausea and vomiting, altered bowel or urinary habits, bloating, pelvic or rectal pressure, and unusual fatigue, irritability, or depression.

Then obtain a menstrual and sexual history. Ask the patient if her menstrual flow is heavy or scant. Have her describe any vaginal discharge between menses. Does she experience pain during sexual intercourse, and does it occur with menses? Find out what relieves her cramps. Does she take pain medication? Is it effective? Note her method of contraception, and ask about a history of pelvic infection. Does she have signs or symptoms of urinary system obstruction, such as pyuria, urine retention, or incontinence? Determine how she copes with stress.

Physical assessment

Perform a focused physical examination. Inspect the abdomen for distention, and palpate for tenderness and masses. Note costovertebral angle tenderness.

Analysis

Dysmenorrhea may be idiopathic, as in premenstrual syndrome and primary dysmenorrhea. It commonly results from endometriosis and other pelvic disorders. It may also result from structural abnormalities, such as an imperforate hymen. Stress and poor health may

(Text continues on page 188.)

Female GU system: Interpreting your findings

After you assess the patient, a group of findings may lead you to suspect a particular disorder. The chart below shows common groups of findings for the signs and symptoms of the female genitourinary (GU) system, along with their probable causes.

Sign or symptom and findings	Probable cause
Pain	
• Steady, aching pain that begins before menses and peaks at the height of menstrual flow (dysmenorrhea); pain may also occur between menstrual periods • Pain may radiate to the perineum or rectum • Premenstrual spotting • Dyspareunia • Infertility • Nausea and vomiting • Tender, fixed adnexal mass palpable on bimanual examination	Endometriosis
• Severe abdominal pain • Fever • Malaise • Foul-smelling, purulent vaginal discharge • Menorrhagia • Cervical motion tenderness and bilateral adnexal tenderness on pelvic examination	Pelvic inflammatory disease
• Cramping pain that begins with menstrual flow and diminishes with decreasing flow (dysmenorrhea) • Abdominal bloating • Breast tenderness • Depression • Irritability • Headache • Diarrhea	Premenstrual syndrome
Dysuria	
• Urinary frequency • Nocturia • Straining to void • Hematuria • Perineal or low-back pain • Fatigue • Low-grade fever	Cystitis

Female GU system: Interpreting your findings (continued)

Sign or symptom and findings	Probable cause
Dysuria (continued)	
• Dysuria throughout voiding • Bladder distention • Diminished urinary stream • Urinary frequency and urgency • Sensation of bloating or fullness in the lower abdomen or groin	Urinary system obstruction
• Urinary urgency • Hematuria • Cloudy urine • Bladder spasms • Feeling of warmth or burning during urination	Urinary tract infection
Urinary incontinence	
• Urge or overflow incontinence • Hematuria • Dysuria • Nocturia • Urinary frequency • Suprapubic pain from bladder spasms • Palpable mass on bimanual examination	Bladder cancer
• Overflow incontinence • Painless bladder distention • Episodic diarrhea or constipation • Orthostatic hypotension • Syncope • Dysphagia	Diabetic neuropathy
• Urinary urgency and frequency • Visual problems • Sensory impairment • Constipation • Muscle weakness • Emotional lability	Multiple sclerosis

(continued)

Female GU system: Interpreting your findings (continued)

Sign or symptom and findings	Probable cause
Vaginal discharge	
• Profuse, white, curdlike discharge with a yeasty, sweet odor • Exudate may be lightly attached to the labia and vaginal walls • Vulvar redness and edema • Intense labial itching and burning	Candidiasis
• Yellow, mucopurulent, odorless, or acrid discharge • Dysuria • Dyspareunia • Vaginal bleeding after douching or coitus	*Chlamydia* infection
• Yellow or green, foul-smelling discharge that can be expressed from the Bartholin's or Skene's ducts • Dysuria • Urinary frequency and incontinence • Vaginal redness and swelling	Gonorrhea

aggravate dysmenorrhea; rest and mild exercise may relieve it.

PEDIATRIC TIP

Dysmenorrhea is rare during the first year of menses, before the cycle becomes ovulatory. However, generally, more adolescents experience dysmenorrhea than older women.

If the patient is an adolescent, teach her about dysmenorrhea. Dispel myths about it, and inform her that it's a common medical problem. Encourage good hygiene, nutrition, and exercise.

DYSURIA

Dysuria—painful or difficult urination—is commonly accompanied by urinary frequency, urgency, or hesitancy. This symptom usually reflects lower urinary tract infection (UTI)—a common disorder, especially in women.

History

If the patient complains of dysuria, have her describe its severity and location. When did she first notice it? Did anything precipitate it? Does anything aggravate or alleviate it?

Next, ask about previous UTIs or genital infections. Has the patient recently undergone an invasive procedure, such as a cystoscopy or urethral dilatation? Also, ask if she has a history of intestinal disease. Ask about menstrual disorders and use of products that irritate the urinary tract, such as bubble bath salts, feminine deodorants, contraceptive gels, or perineal lotions. Also ask about vaginal discharge or pruritus.

Physical assessment

During the physical examination, inspect the urethral meatus for discharge, irritation, or other abnormalities. A pelvic or rectal examination may be necessary.

Analysis

Dysuria results from lower urinary tract irritation or inflammation, which stimulates nerve endings in the bladder and urethra. The pain's onset provides clues to its cause—for example, pain just before voiding usually indicates bladder irritation or distention, whereas pain at the start of urination typically results from bladder outlet irritation. Pain at the end of voiding may indicate bladder spasms or vaginal candidiasis.

GERIATRIC TIP

Be aware that elderly patients tend to under-report their symptoms, even though postmenopausal women are more likely to experience noninfectious dysuria.

URINARY INCONTINENCE

Incontinence, the uncontrollable passage of urine, results from either a bladder abnormality or a neurologic disorder. A common urologic sign, incontinence may be transient or permanent and may involve large volumes of urine or scant dribbling.

History

Ask the patient when she first noticed the incontinence and whether it began suddenly or gradually. Have her describe her typical urinary pattern: Does incontinence usually occur during the day or at night? Does she have any urinary control, or is she totally incontinent? If she sometimes urinates with control, ask her the usual times and amounts voided. Determine her normal fluid intake. Ask about other urinary problems, such as hesitancy, frequency, urgency, nocturia, and decreased force or interruption of the urinary stream. Also ask if she has ever sought treatment for incontinence or found a way to deal with it herself.

Obtain a medical history, especially noting UTI, childbirth, spinal injury or tumor, cerebrovascular accident, or surgery involving the bladder or pelvic floor.

Physical assessment

After completing the history, have the patient empty her bladder. Inspect the urethral meatus for obvious inflammation or anatomic defect. Have her bear down; note any urine leakage. Gently palpate the abdomen for bladder distention, which signals urine retention. Perform a complete neurologic assessment, noting motor and sensory function and obvious muscle atrophy.

Analysis

Urinary incontinence can be classified as stress, overflow, urge, or total incontinence. Stress incontinence refers to intermittent leakage resulting from a sudden physical strain, such as a cough, sneeze, or quick movement. Overflow incontinence is a dribble resulting from urine retention, which fills the bladder and prevents it from contracting with sufficient force to expel a urinary stream. Urge incontinence refers to the inability to suppress a sudden urge to urinate. Total incontinence is continuous leakage resulting from the bladder's inability to retain any urine.

PEDIATRIC TIP

Causes of incontinence in children include infrequent or incomplete voiding. These may also lead to UTI. Ectopic ureteral orifice is an uncommon congenital anomaly associated with incontinence. A complete diagnostic evaluation is usually necessary to rule out organic disease.

GERIATRIC TIP

Diagnosing a UTI in elderly patients can be problematic because many come in only with urinary incontinence or changes in mental status, anorexia, or malaise. In addition, many elderly patients without UTIs come in with dysuria, frequency, urgency, or incontinence.

VAGINAL DISCHARGE

Common in women of childbearing age, physiologic vaginal discharge is mucoid, clear or white, nonbloody, and odorless. Produced by the cervical mucosa and, to a lesser degree, by the vulvar glands, this discharge may occasionally be scant or profuse due to estrogenic stimulation and changes during menses. However, a marked increase in discharge or a change in discharge color, odor, or consistency can signal disease.

History

Ask the patient to describe the onset, color, consistency, odor, and texture of her vaginal discharge. How does the discharge differ from her usual vaginal secretions? Is the onset related to her menstrual cycle? Also, ask about associated symptoms, such as dysuria and perineal pruritus and burning. Does she have spotting after coitus or douching? Ask about recent changes in sexual habits and hygiene practices. Is she or could she be pregnant? Next, ask if she has had vaginal discharge before or has ever been treated for a vaginal infection. What treatment was given? Did she complete the course of medication? Ask about current use of medications, especially antibiotics, oral estrogens, and contraceptives.

Physical assessment

Examine the external genitalia and note the character of the discharge. Observe vulvar and vaginal tissues for redness, edema, and excoriation. Palpate the inguinal lymph nodes to detect tenderness or enlargement, and palpate the abdomen for tenderness. A pelvic examination may be required. Obtain vaginal discharge specimens for testing.

Analysis

The discharge may result from an infection, a sexually transmitted or reproductive tract disease, a fistula, or use of certain drugs. In addition, the prolonged presence of a foreign body, such as a tampon or diaphragm, in the patient's vagina can cause irritation and an inflammatory exudate, as can frequent douching, feminine hygiene products, contraceptive products, bubble baths, and colored or perfumed toilet papers.

PEDIATRIC TIP

Female neonates who have been exposed to maternal estrogens in utero may have a white mucous vaginal discharge for the first month after birth; a yellow mucous discharge indicates a pathologic condition. In the older child, a purulent, foul-smelling, and bloody vaginal discharge may result if a foreign object is placed in the vagina. The possibility of sexual abuse should also be considered.

GERIATRIC TIP

The postmenopausal vaginal mucosa becomes thin due to decreased estrogen levels. Together with a rise in vaginal pH, this reduces resistance to infectious agents, increasing the incidence of vaginitis.

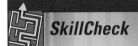

SkillCheck

1. What is the leading cause of lost time from school and work among women of childbearing age?
   a. Urinary incontinence
   b. Dysuria
   c. Dysmenorrhea
   d. Vaginal discharge

Answer: c. Dysmenorrhea is the leading cause; it affects over 50% of menstruating women.

2. What should urinary incontinence resulting from a cough or sneeze be classified as?
   a. Stress incontinence
   b. Overflow incontinence
   c. Urge incontinence
   d. Total incontinence

Answer: a. Stress incontinence refers to intermittent leakage resulting from a sudden physical strain, such as a cough or sneeze.

3. Dysuria is usually a symptom of which common disorder?
   a. Bladder cancer
   b. Cystitis
   c. Pyelonephritis
   d. Lower UTI

Answer: d. Lower UTI is commonly associated with dysuria, urinary frequency, urgency, or hesitancy.

4. How does physiologic vaginal discharge usually appear?
   a. Mucoid, clear, or white; nonbloody; and odorless
   b. White, curdlike, and profuse with a yeasty odor
   c. Yellow or green and foul smelling
   d. Frothy, greenish yellow, and profuse

Answer: a. Mucoid—discharge that's clear or white and nonbloody and odorless is produced by the cervical mucosa and vulvar glands. It may be scant or profuse due to estrogenic stimulation and changes during menses.

5. In which population of people is it possible for both kidneys to be palpable?
   a. Children
   b. Elderly people
   c. Women of childbearing age
   d. Men of any age

Answer: b. Elderly people have decreased muscle tone and elasticity, so you may be able to palpate both kidneys.

Male genitourinary system

A disorder of the male urinary or reproductive system can have far-reaching consequences. Besides affecting the system itself, such disorders can trigger problems in other body systems. It also can affect the patient's quality of life, self-esteem, and sense of well-being.

Despite these implications, many men are reluctant to discuss their problems with a nurse or to have intimate areas of their bodies examined. Your challenge, then, is to perform a 3-minute assessment that's both skilled and sensitive. To do this, be aware of your own feelings about sexuality. If you appear comfortable discussing the patient's problem, he'll be encouraged to talk openly as well.

This chapter presents a review of the anatomy and physiology and physical assessment techniques for the male genitourinary (GU) system, along with 3-minute assessment guidelines for common signs and symptoms associated with the male GU system.

Anatomy and physiology

A quick, thorough, and accurate assessment of the male GU system requires an understanding of the organs and structures of the urinary and reproductive systems and the way they work.

URINARY SYSTEM

The urinary system helps maintain homeostasis by regulating fluid and electrolyte balance. It consists of the kidneys, ureters, bladder, and urethra. The essential functions of the system, forming urine and maintaining homeostasis, occur in the highly vascular kidneys. For more information about the urinary system, see chapter 11, Female genitourinary system.

The male and female urinary systems function in the same way, although a man's urethra is about 6″ (15 cm) longer than a woman's, because it must pass through the erectile tissue of the penis.

REPRODUCTIVE SYSTEM

In men, the urethra is also part of the reproductive system, carrying semen as well as urine. The male reproductive system also includes the penis, scrotum, testicles, epididymis, vas deferens, seminal vesicles, and prostate gland. (See *Male reproductive system.*)

The penis consists of the shaft, glans, urethral meatus, corona, and prepuce. The skin of the penis is hairless and usually darker than the skin on other parts of the body.

The shaft contains three columns of vascular erectile tissue. The glans is lo-

A CLOSER LOOK

Male reproductive system

This illustration shows the important structures of the male reproductive system.

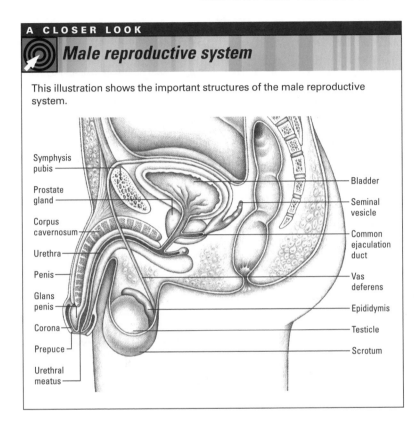

- Symphysis pubis
- Prostate gland
- Corpus cavernosum
- Urethra
- Penis
- Glans penis
- Corona
- Prepuce
- Urethral meatus

- Bladder
- Seminal vesicle
- Common ejaculation duct
- Vas deferens
- Epididymis
- Testicle
- Scrotum

cated at the end of the penis. The urethral meatus, a slitlike opening, is normally located ventrally at the tip of the glans. The corona is formed by the junction of the glans and the shaft. The prepuce, the loose skin covering the glans, is commonly removed shortly after birth by a surgical procedure called *circumcision.*

When the penile tissues are engorged with blood, the erect penis can discharge sperm. During sexual activity, sperm and semen are forcefully ejaculated from the urethral meatus.

The scrotum is located at the base of the penis. It's a loose, wrinkled, deeply pigmented pouch that consists of a muscle layer covered by skin. Each of its two compartments contains a testicle, epididymis, and portions of the spermatic cord. The left side of the scrotum is usually lower than the right because the left spermatic cord is longer.

The testicles are oval, rubbery structures suspended vertically and slightly forward in the scrotum. They produce testosterone and sperm.

Testosterone stimulates the changes that occur during puberty, which starts between age 9½ and 13½. The testicles enlarge, pubic hair grows, and penis size increases. Secondary sex characteristics appear, such as facial and body hair, muscle development, and voice changes.

The epididymis is a reservoir for maturing sperm. It curves over the posterolateral surface of each testicle, creating a visible bulge on the surface. In a small number of men, the epididymis is located anteriorly.

The vas deferens—a storage site and the pathway for sperm—begins at the lower end of the epididymis, climbs the spermatic cord, travels through the inguinal canal, and ends in the abdominal cavity where it rests on the fundus of the bladder.

A pair of saclike glands, the seminal vesicles are found on the lower posterior surface of the bladder in front of the rectum. Secretions from the seminal vesicles help form seminal fluid.

The prostate is a walnut-shaped gland, about 1½″ (4 cm) in diameter, that surrounds the urethra like a doughnut, just below the bladder. It produces a thin, milky, alkaline fluid that mixes with seminal fluid during ejaculation to enhance sperm activity.

Physical assessment

To perform a physical assessment of the male GU system, use inspection, percussion, palpation, and auscultation. Assessment of the urinary system may be done now or as part of the GI assessment. (See *Male GU system: Normal findings.*)

EXAMINING THE URINARY SYSTEM

In many ways, assessing the male urinary system is similar to assessing the female urinary system. Before performing an assessment, ask the patient to urinate; then help him into the supine position with his arms at his sides. As you proceed, expose only the areas being examined.

Inspection

First, inspect the patient's abdomen. When he's in a supine position, his abdomen should be smooth, flat or concave, and symmetrical. The skin should be free from lesions, bruises, discoloration, and prominent veins.

Look for abdominal distention. Tight, glistening skin and striae—silvery streaks—are caused by rapidly developing skin tension. These are signs of ascites, which may accompany nephrotic syndrome. This syndrome is characterized by edema, increased urine protein levels, and decreased serum albumin levels.

Percussion

First, tell the patient what you're going to do; otherwise, he may be startled by your touch, and you could mistake his reaction for a feeling of acute tenderness. While the patient is lying down, percuss the bladder to elicit tenderness or dullness. To perform indirect fist percussion, ask the patient to sit up with his back to you. Percuss the kidneys, checking for pain or tenderness, which suggests kidney infection. Place one hand at the costovertebral angle and strike it with the ulnar surface of your other hand.

Remember to percuss both sides of the body to assess both kidneys and

CHECKLIST
Male GU system: Normal findings

Inspection
❏ Abdomen is symmetrical and smooth, and flat or concave when the patient is in a supine position.
❏ Skin is free from lesions, bruises, discoloration, and prominent veins.
❏ No abdominal distention or edema is apparent.
❏ Penis appears slightly wrinkled, with the color ranging from pink to dark brown, depending on the patient's skin color.
❏ Smegma may be present.
❏ Urethral meatus is pink and smooth and located in the center of the glans.
❏ Scrotum is free from swelling and edema but may have some sebaceous cysts.
❏ Pubic area is free from lesions and parasites.

Percussion
❏ No costovertebral angle tenderness is detectable.

❏ Tympany is heard over the empty bladder.

Palpation
❏ Kidneys are unpalpable, except in very thin or elderly patients.
❏ Bladder is unpalpable.
❏ Penis feels somewhat firm, with the skin smooth and movable.
❏ Testicles are equally sized, move freely in the scrotal sac, and feel firm, smooth, and rubbery.
❏ Epididymis is smooth, discrete, nontender, and free from swelling and induration.
❏ No inguinal or femoral hernias are apparent.
❏ Prostate gland is smooth and rubbery, is about the size of a walnut, and doesn't protrude into the rectal lumen.

Auscultation
❏ No bruits can be heard over the renal arteries.

percuss the abdomen to assess the bladder for tenderness and fullness. A dull sound instead of the normal tympany may indicate retained urine in the bladder, caused by bladder dysfunction or infection. You also can palpate the bladder to check for distention. Because the kidneys aren't usually palpable, detecting an enlarged kidney should be investigated with further tests. Kidney enlargement may accompany hydronephrosis, a cyst, or a tumor.

Auscultation
Auscultate the upper abdomen or costovertebral angle to assess the renal arteries to rule out bruits, which signal renal artery stenosis. You can do this now or as part of an abdominal assessment.

EXAMINING THE REPRODUCTIVE SYSTEM
Before examining the reproductive system, explain what you are going to do and put on gloves. Make the patient as comfortable as possible to help the patient feel less embarrassed.

Inspection
Gently inspect the penis, scrotum, and testicles as well as the inguinal and femoral areas.

Start by examining the penis. Penis size depends on the patient's age and overall development. The penile skin should be slightly wrinkled and pink to light brown in white patients and light brown to dark brown in black patients. Check the penile shaft and glans for lesions, nodules, inflammation, and swelling. Also check the glans for smegma, a cheesy secretion commonly found beneath the prepuce. A male patient who is obese may appear to have an abnormally small penis. You may have to retract the fat over the symphysis pubis to properly assess the penis.

Then gently compress the tip of the glans to open the urethral meatus. It should be located in the center of the glans and be pink and smooth. If the meatus is not centered, the patient may have hypospadias. Inspect it for swelling, discharge, lesions, inflammation and, especially, genital warts. If you note discharge, obtain a culture specimen.

Have the patient hold his penis away from his scrotum so you can observe the scrotum's general size and appearance. The skin here is darker than on the rest of the body. Spread the surface of the scrotum, and examine the skin for nodules, redness, ulceration, and distended veins.

Sebaceous cysts—firm, white to yellow, nontender cutaneous lesions—are a normal finding. Also, check for scrotal edema, which may be a sign of cardiovascular disease. Spread the pubic hair and check the skin for lesions and parasites. If you see an enlarged scrotum in a boy younger than age 2, suspect a scrotal extension of an inguinal hernia, a hydrocele, or both.

Palpation

Palpate the penis, testicles, epididymis, spermatic cords, inguinal and femoral areas, and prostate gland.

Use your thumb and forefinger to palpate the entire penile shaft. It should be somewhat firm, and the skin should be smooth and movable. Note swelling, nodules, or indurations.

Gently palpate both testicles between your thumb and first two fingers. Assess their size, shape, and response to pressure. A normal response is a deep visceral pain. The testicles should be equal in size, move freely in the scrotal sac, and feel firm, smooth, and rubbery.

If you note hard, irregular areas or lumps, transilluminate them by darkening the room and pressing the head of a flashlight against the scrotum, behind the lump. The testicle and any lumps, masses, warts, or blood-filled areas will appear as opaque shadows.

Transilluminate the other testicle to compare your findings. This is also a good time to reinforce the methods and importance of doing a monthly testicular self-examination.

Next, palpate the epididymis, which is usually located in the posterolateral area of the testicle. It should be smooth, discrete, nontender, and free from swelling and induration.

Palpate both spermatic cords, which are located above each testicle. Palpate from the base of the epididymis to the inguinal canal. The vas deferens is a smooth, movable cord inside the spermatic cord. If you feel swelling, irregularity, or nodules, transilluminate the problem area, as described above. If serous fluid is present, you won't see this glow.

Have the patient stand. Then ask him to hold his breath and bear down while you inspect the inguinal and femoral areas for bulges or hernias. A hernia is a loop of bowel that comes through a muscle wall.

To assess the patient for a direct inguinal hernia, place two fingers over each external inguinal ring, and ask him to bear down. If he has a hernia, you'll feel a bulge.

To assess the patient for an indirect inguinal hernia, examine him while he's standing and then while he's in a supine position with his knee flexed on the side you're examining. (See *Palpating for an indirect inguinal hernia.*)

Place your index finger on the neck of the scrotum, and gently push upward into the inguinal canal. When you've inserted your finger as far as possible, ask the patient to bear down or cough. A hernia feels like a mass of tissue that withdraws when it meets the finger.

Although you can't palpate the femoral canal, you can estimate its location to help detect a femoral hernia. Place your right index finger on the right femoral artery with your finger pointing toward the patient's head. Keep your other fingers close together. Your middle finger will rest on the femoral vein; your ring finger, on the femoral canal. Note tenderness or masses. Use your left hand to check the patient's left side.

Before examining the prostate, warn the patient that he'll feel some pressure or urgency during this examination. Have him stand and lean over the examination table. If he can't do this, have him lie on his left side, with his right knee and hip flexed or with both knees drawn toward his chest. Inspect the skin of the perineal, anal, and pos-

Palpating for an indirect inguinal hernia

To palpate for an indirect inguinal hernia, place your gloved finger on the neck of the scrotum, and insert the finger into the inguinal canal, as shown. Then ask the patient to bear down.

If the patient has a hernia, you'll feel a soft mass at your fingertip.

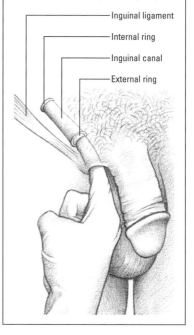

Inguinal ligament

Internal ring

Inguinal canal

External ring

terior scrotal areas. It should be smooth and unbroken, with no protruding masses.

Then lubricate the gloved index finger of your dominant hand. Tell the patient to relax to ease the passage of your finger and insert it into the rectum through the anal sphincter. With your

Palpating the prostate gland

To palpate the prostate gland, insert your gloved, lubricated index finger into the rectum. Then palpate the prostate on the anterior rectal wall, just past the anorectal ring, as shown.

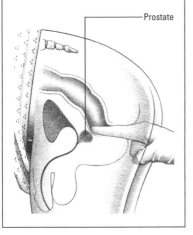

Prostate

finger pad, palpate the prostate gland on the anterior rectal wall just past the anorectal ring. The gland should feel smooth, rubbery, and about the size of a walnut. (See *Palpating the prostate gland*.)

If the prostate gland protrudes into the rectal lumen, it's probably enlarged. An enlarged prostate gland is classified from grade 1 (protruding less than ⅜″ [1 cm] into the rectal lumen) to grade 4 (protruding more than 1¼″ [3 cm] into the rectal lumen). Also, note tenderness or nodules.

Guidelines for a 3-minute assessment

If your patient reports having a problem that involves the urinary or reproductive system, you should proceed with a 3-minute assessment. Begin your assessment by making some general observations and taking the patient's vital signs. Then focus on the patient's chief sign or symptom.

MAKING GENERAL OBSERVATIONS
Your general observations should include noting the patient's overall appearance and skin condition.

Overall appearance
Look for signs of fluid imbalance, such as dry mucous membranes, sunken eyeballs, edema, or ascites. Observe the patient for signs of pain such as guarding or splinting his abdomen, grimacing, or shifting positions frequently.

Skin condition
Observe the patient's skin. A person with decreased renal function may be pale because of a low hemoglobin level or may even have uremic frost—snowlike crystals on the skin from metabolic wastes.

CHECKING VITAL SIGNS
The patient's vital signs and weight can offer important information. For example, a patient's vital signs

might reveal hypertension, which can cause renal dysfunction if it's uncontrolled. Check blood pressure in each arm. Take his temperature, noting fever and accompanying chills. Weighing the patient can provide information about fluid status and is important for patients with urinary disorders or renal failure, especially those receiving dialysis.

FOCUSING ON THE CHIEF SIGN OR SYMPTOM

After you've made general observations and checked the patient's vital signs, you'll want to focus on the chief GU sign or symptom for the history and physical assessment.

Further assessment

Organs and structures outside of the male GU system may need assessment to determine the cause of the symptom. For example, an abdominal assessment may be performed when a patient seeks care for scrotal swelling. Additionally, pitting scrotal edema could be a sign of cardiovascular disease, making an assessment of this system necessary. After you've obtained the necessary information about the patient's chief sign or symptom and completed your physical assessment, you'll begin to formulate a diagnostic impression. (See *Male GU system: Interpreting your findings*, pages 200 to 202.)

Common signs and symptoms

A man may seek care for a number of signs and symptoms related to the GU system. Some common ones are male genital lesions, scrotal swelling, urethral discharge, collicky flank pain, and urinary hesitancy.

MALE GENITAL LESIONS

Among the diverse lesions that may affect the male genitalia are warts, papules, ulcers, scales, and pustules. These common lesions may be painful or painless, singular or multiple. They may be limited to the genitalia or may also occur elsewhere on the body.

History

Begin by asking the patient when he first noticed the lesion. Did it erupt after he began taking a new drug or after a trip out of the country? Next, take a complete sexual history, noting the frequency of relations and the number of sexual partners. Has he had similar lesions before? If so, did he get medical treatment for them? Find out if he has been treating the lesion himself. If so, how? Does the lesion itch? If so, is the itching constant or does it bother him only at night? Note whether the lesion is painful or has drainage.

Physical assessment

Before you examine the patient, observe his clothing. Do his pants fit properly? Tight pants or underwear, especially those made of nonabsorbent fabrics, can promote the growth of bacteria and fungi. Examine the entire skin surface, noting the location, size, color,

Male GU system: Interpreting your findings

After you assess the patient, a group of findings may lead you to suspect a particular disorder. The chart below shows common groups of findings for the signs and symptoms of the male genitourinary (GU) system, along with their probable causes.

Sign or symptom and findings	Probable cause
Male genital lesions	
• Fluid-filled vesicles on the glans penis, foreskin, or penile shaft • Painful ulcers • Tender inguinal lymph nodes • Fever • Malaise • Dysuria	Genital herpes
• Painless warts (tiny pink swellings that grow and become pedunculated) near the urethral meatus • Lesions spread to the perineum and the perianal area • Cauliflower appearance of multiple swellings	Genital warts
• Sharply defined, slightly raised, scaling patches on the inner thigh or groin (bilaterally), or on the scrotum or penis • Severe pruritus	Tinea cruris (jock itch)
Scrotal swelling	
• Swollen scrotum that's soft or unusually firm • Bowel sounds may be auscultated in the scrotum • Sharp, steady groin pain that increases with tension or straining may occur with an inguinal hernia • Swelling in the groin area occurs with an inguinal hernia.	Hernia

and pattern of the lesions. Do genital lesions resemble those on other parts of the body? Palpate for nodules, masses, and tenderness. Also, look for bleeding, edema, or signs of infection such as erythema.

Male GU system: Interpreting your findings (continued)

Sign or symptom and findings	Probable cause
Scrotal swelling (continued)	
• Gradual scrotal swelling • Scrotum may be soft and cystic or firm and tense • Painless • Round, nontender scrotal mass on palpation • Glowing when transilluminated	Hydrocele
• Scrotal swelling with sudden and severe pain • Unilateral elevation of the affected testicle • Nausea and vomiting	Testicular torsion
Urethral discharge	
• Purulent or milky urethral discharge • Sudden fever and chills • Lower back pain • Myalgia • Perineal fullness • Arthralgia • Urinary frequency and urgency • Cloudy urine • Dysuria • Tense, boggy, very tender, and warm prostate palpated on digital rectal examination	Prostatitis
• Opaque, gray, yellowish, or blood-tinged discharge that's painless • Dysuria • Eventual anuria	Urethral neoplasm
• Scant or profuse urethral discharge that's either thin and clear, mucoid, or thick and purulent • Urinary hesitancy, frequency, and urgency • Dysuria • Itching and burning around the meatus	Urethritis

(continued)

Analysis

Genital lesions may result from infection, neoplasms, parasites, allergy, or the use of certain drugs. These lesions can profoundly affect the patient's self-image. In fact, the patient may hesitate to seek medical attention because he fears cancer or sexually transmitted disease (STD).

Genital lesions that arise from an STD could mean that the patient is at risk for human immunodeficiency virus

Male GU system: Interpreting your findings (continued)

Sign or symptom and findings	Probable cause
Urinary hesitancy	
• Reduced caliber and force of urinary stream • Perineal pain • A feeling of incomplete voiding • Inability to stop the urine stream • Urinary frequency • Urinary incontinence • Bladder distention	Benign prostatic hyperplasia
• Urinary frequency and dribbling • Nocturia • Dysuria • Bladder distention • Perineal pain • Constipation • Hard, nodular prostate palpated on digital rectal examination	Prostatic cancer
• Dysuria • Urinary frequency and urgency • Hematuria • Cloudy urine • Bladder spasms • Costovertebral angle tenderness • Suprapubic, low back, pelvic, or flank pain • Urethral discharge	Urinary tract infection

(HIV). Genital ulcers make HIV transmission between sexual partners more likely. Unfortunately, if the patient is treating himself, he may alter the lesions, making differential diagnosis especially difficult.

PEDIATRIC TIP
In infants, contact dermatitis ("diaper rash") may produce minor irritation or bright red, weepy, excoriated lesions. Use of disposable diapers and careful cleaning of the penis and scrotum can help reduce diaper rash.

In children, impetigo may cause pustules with thick, yellow, weepy crusts. Like adults, children may develop genital warts, but they'll need more reassurance that the treatment (excision) won't hurt or castrate them. Children with an STD must be evaluated for signs of sexual abuse.

Adolescents ages 15 to 19 have a high incidence of STDs and related genital lesions. Syphilis, however, may also be congenital.

GERIATRIC TIP
Elderly adults who are sexually active with multiple partners have as high a risk of developing an STD as do younger adults. However, because of

decreased immunity, poor hygiene, poor symptom reporting, and possibly several concurrent conditions, they may seek treatment for different symptoms. Seborrheic dermatitis lasts longer and is more extensive in bedridden patients and those with Parkinson's disease.

SCROTAL SWELLING

Scrotal swelling occurs when a condition affecting the testicles, epididymis, or scrotal skin produces edema or a mass; the penis may or may not be involved. Scrotal swelling may also occur as a symptom of a systemic disease causing fluid retention. Scrotal swelling may affect males of any age; it can be unilateral or bilateral and painful or painless.

History

If the patient isn't in distress, proceed with the history. Ask about injury to the scrotum, urethral discharge, cloudy urine, increased urinary frequency, and dysuria. Ask him if he has experienced groin pain with lifting or straining. Has he noticed any lump in the groin area? Is the patient sexually active? When was his last sexual contact? Find out about recent illnesses, particularly mumps. Does he have a history of prostate surgery or prolonged catheterization? Does changing his body position or level of activity affect the swelling?

Physical assessment

Palpate the patient's abdomen for tenderness and inguinal lumps or signs of a hernia. Then examine the entire genital area. Assess the scrotum with the patient in supine and standing positions. Note its size and color. Is the swelling unilateral or bilateral? Do you see signs of trauma or bruising? Gently palpate the scrotum for a cyst or a lump. Note especially tenderness or increased firmness. Check the position of the testicles in the scrotum. Finally, transilluminate the scrotum to distinguish a fluid-filled cyst from a solid mass. (A solid mass can't be transilluminated.)

Analysis

Scrotal swelling can result from inguinal hernia, hydrocele, or trauma to the scrotum. The sudden onset of painful scrotal swelling suggests torsion of a testicle or testicular appendages, especially in a prepubescent male. This emergency requires immediate surgery to untwist and stabilize the spermatic cord or to remove the appendage.

PEDIATRIC TIP

A thorough physical assessment is especially important for children with scrotal swelling, who may be unable to offer clues about their medical history. In children up to age 1, a hernia or hydrocele of the spermatic cord may stem from abnormal fetal development. In infants, scrotal swelling may stem from ammonia-related dermatitis, if diapers aren't changed often enough. In prepubescent males, it usually results from torsion of the spermatic cord.

Other disorders that can produce scrotal swelling in children include epididymitis (rare in those younger than age 10), traumatic orchitis from contact sports, and mumps, which usually occurs after puberty.

URETHRAL DISCHARGE

Discharge from the urinary meatus may be purulent, mucoid, or thin; sanguineous or clear; and scant or profuse. It usually develops suddenly.

History

Ask the patient when he first noticed the discharge, and have him describe its color, consistency, and quantity. Does the patient have pain on urination? Does he have difficulty initiating a urinary stream? Ask the patient about other associated signs and symptoms, such as fever, chills, and perineal fullness. Explore his history for prostate problems, STD, or urinary tract infection (UTI). Ask the patient if he has had recent sexual contacts or a new sexual partner.

Physical assessment

Inspect the patient's urethral meatus for inflammation and swelling. Using proper technique, obtain a culture specimen. Then obtain a urine sample for urinalysis and possibly a three-glass urine sample. The prostate gland may have to be palpated.

Analysis

Urethral discharge is most common in men with a prostate infection and certain STDs. Other causes may include urethral neoplasm, a rare cancer, and urethritis, an inflammatory disorder that can be sexually transmitted.

PEDIATRIC TIP

Carefully evaluate a child with urethral discharge for evidence of sexual and physical abuse.

GERIATRIC TIP

Urethral discharge in elderly males isn't usually related to an STD.

URINARY HESITANCY

Hesitancy—difficulty starting a urinary stream—usually arises gradually, often going unnoticed until urine retention causes bladder distention and discomfort.

History

Ask the patient when he first noticed hesitancy and whether he has ever had the problem before. Ask about other urinary problems, especially reduced force or interruption of the urinary stream. Ask if he has ever been treated for a prostate problem or UTI or obstruction. Obtain a drug history.

Physical assessment

Inspect the patient's urethral meatus for inflammation, discharge, and other abnormalities. Examine the anal sphincter, and test sensation in the perineum. Obtain a clean-catch sample for urinalysis. Palpate the prostate gland.

Analysis

Hesitancy can result from a UTI, a partial lower urinary tract obstruction, a neuromuscular disorder, or use of certain drugs. Occurring at all ages and in both sexes, it's most common in older men with prostatic enlargement.

PEDIATRIC TIP

The most common cause of urinary obstruction in male infants is posterior strictures in the prostatic urethra. Infants with this problem may have a less forceful urinary stream and may also present with fever caused by a UTI, failure to thrive, or a palpable bladder.

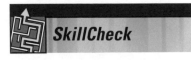

SkillCheck

1. Which disorder is an emergency requiring immediate surgery?
   a. Inguinal hernia
   b. Hydrocele
   c. Testicular torsion
   d. Testicular tumor

Answer: c. Testicular torsion is an emergency that requires immediate surgery to untwist and stabilize the spermatic cord or to remove the appendage.

2. What's the characteristic sign of testicular torsion?
   a. Urinary hesitancy
   b. Urethral discharge
   c. Penile lesion
   d. Scrotal swelling

Answer: d. Sudden scrotal swelling and severe pain signal testicular torsion. Nausea and vomiting may also occur.

3. Urethral discharge is most common in patients with:
   a. bladder cancer.
   b. a UTI.
   c. a prostate infection.
   d. a urethral neoplasm.

Answer: c. Men with a prostate infection will commonly experience urethral discharge.

4. How should the prostate feel on digital rectal examination?
   a. About the size of a walnut
   b. Like it protrudes into the rectal lumen
   c. Smooth with some nodules present
   d. Very tender to the patient

Answer: a. The prostate should feel smooth, rubbery, and about the size of a walnut.

5. Although the male and female urinary systems function in the same way, there's a difference in the length of the:
   a. urethra.
   b. ureter.
   c. bladder.
   d. epididymis.

Answer: a. Because a man's urethra passes through the erectile tissue of the penis, it's about 6″ (15 cm) longer than a woman's.

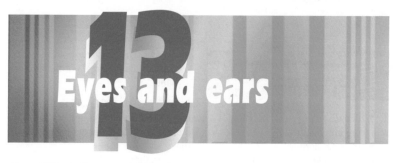

Eyes and ears

About 70% of all sensory information reaches the brain through the eyes. Disorders in vision can interfere with a patient's ability to function independently, perceive the world, and enjoy beauty. Similarly, hearing allows us to communicate with others. Because these senses play such vital roles in daily life, problems should be evaluated quickly.

A rapid, thorough assessment of your patient's eyes and ears can help you identify problems that can affect the patient's health and quality of life. This chapter provides you with a review of the anatomy and physiology of the eyes and ears, basic physical assessment techniques, and 3-minute assessment guidelines to evaluate common problems with vision or hearing.

Anatomy and physiology

To perform an accurate physical assessment, you need to understand the anatomy and physiology of the eyes and ears.

EYE STRUCTURES

The eyes are delicate sensory organs equipped with many protective structures. On the outside, the bony orbits protect the eye from trauma. Eyelids (or palpebrae), lashes, and the lacrimal apparatus protect the eyes from injury, dust, and foreign bodies. (See *Structures of the eye.*)

Sclera, choroid, and vitreous humor

The white coating on the outside of the eyeball, the sclera, maintains the eye's size and shape. The pigmented, vascular choroid, which lines the recessed portion of the eyeball beneath the sclera, contains a network of arteries and veins that maintain blood supply to the eye. The vitreous humor is a thick, gelatinous material that fills the space directly behind the lens and maintains the retina's placement and the eyeball's spherical shape.

Bulbar conjunctiva and cornea

The bulbar conjunctiva is a thin, transparent membrane that lines the eyelids and covers and protects the anterior portion of the white sclera. The cornea is a smooth, avascular, transparent tissue that merges with the sclera at the limbus. It refracts, or bends, light rays entering the eye.

The cornea, which is located in front of the pupil and iris, is fed by the ophthalmic branch of cranial nerve V (the trigeminal nerve). Stimulation of this nerve initiates a protective blink, the corneal reflex.

Structures of the eye

This cross section details important anatomic structures of the eye.

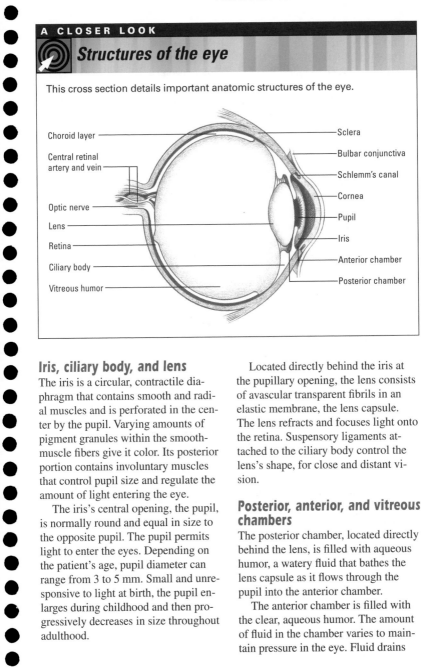

Iris, ciliary body, and lens

The iris is a circular, contractile diaphragm that contains smooth and radial muscles and is perforated in the center by the pupil. Varying amounts of pigment granules within the smooth-muscle fibers give it color. Its posterior portion contains involuntary muscles that control pupil size and regulate the amount of light entering the eye.

The iris's central opening, the pupil, is normally round and equal in size to the opposite pupil. The pupil permits light to enter the eyes. Depending on the patient's age, pupil diameter can range from 3 to 5 mm. Small and unresponsive to light at birth, the pupil enlarges during childhood and then progressively decreases in size throughout adulthood.

Located directly behind the iris at the pupillary opening, the lens consists of avascular transparent fibrils in an elastic membrane, the lens capsule. The lens refracts and focuses light onto the retina. Suspensory ligaments attached to the ciliary body control the lens's shape, for close and distant vision.

Posterior, anterior, and vitreous chambers

The posterior chamber, located directly behind the lens, is filled with aqueous humor, a watery fluid that bathes the lens capsule as it flows through the pupil into the anterior chamber.

The anterior chamber is filled with the clear, aqueous humor. The amount of fluid in the chamber varies to maintain pressure in the eye. Fluid drains from the anterior chamber through collecting channels into Schlemm's canal.

The vitreous chamber, located behind the lens, occupies four-fifths of the eyeball. This chamber is filled with vitreous humor, an avascular gelatinous substance that maintains the shape of the eyeball.

Retina

The innermost region of the eyeball, the retina receives visual stimuli and transmits images to the brain for processing. Four sets of retinal blood vessels—the superonasal, inferonasal, superotemporal, and inferotemporal—are visible through an ophthalmoscope.

Each set of vessels contains a transparent arteriole and vein. As these vessels leave the optic disc, they become progressively thinner, intertwining as they extend to the periphery of the retina.

The optic disc is the opening within the retina's nasal portion through which the ganglion nerve fibers exit to form the optic nerve. This area—a well-defined, round or oval area measuring less than $1/8''$ (0.3 cm)—is called the *blind spot* because no photoreceptors are located there.

The physiologic cup is a light-colored depression within the temporal side of the optic disc where blood vessels enter the retina. It covers one-fourth to one-third of the disc but doesn't extend completely to the margin.

Photoreceptor neurons make up the retina's visual receptors. Not visible through the ophthalmoscope, these receptors—some shaped like rods and some like cones—are responsible for vision. Rods respond to low-intensity light, but they don't provide sharp images or color vision. Cones respond to bright light and provide high-acuity color vision.

Located laterally from the optic disc, the macula is slightly darker than the rest of the retina and contains no visible retinal vessels. Because its borders are poorly defined, the macula is difficult to see on an ophthalmologic examination. It's best identified by having the patient look straight at the ophthalmoscope's light.

The fovea centralis, a slight depression in the macula, appears as a bright reflection when examined with an ophthalmoscope. Because the fovea contains the heaviest concentration of cones, it acts as the eye's clearest vision and color receptor.

Extraocular muscles

Eye movement is controlled by six extraocular muscles that are innervated or stimulated by the cranial nerves. The coordinated actions of those muscles allow the eyes to move in tandem, ensuring clear vision.

EAR STRUCTURES

The ear is divided into three parts: external, middle, and inner. The anatomy and physiology of each part play separate but equally important roles in hearing. (See *Structures of the ear.*)

External ear

The flexible external ear consists mainly of elastic cartilage. This part of the ear contains the ear flap, also known as the *auricle* or *pinna,* and the auditory canal. The outer third of this canal has a bony framework.

Structures of the ear

Use this illustration to review the structures of the ear.

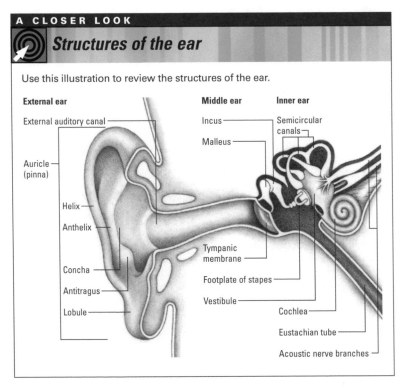

External ear

- External auditory canal
- Auricle (pinna)
- Helix
- Anthelix
- Concha
- Antitragus
- Lobule

Middle ear

- Incus
- Malleus
- Tympanic membrane
- Footplate of stapes
- Vestibule

Inner ear

- Semicircular canals
- Cochlea
- Eustachian tube
- Acoustic nerve branches

Middle ear

The tympanic membrane separates the external and middle ear. This pearl gray structure consists of three layers: skin, fibrous tissue, and a mucous membrane. Its upper portion, the pars flaccida, has little support; its lower portion, the pars tensa, is held taut. The center, or umbo, is attached to the tip of the long process of the malleus on the other side of the tympanic membrane.

A small, air-filled structure, the middle ear performs three vital functions:
- It transmits sound vibrations across the bony ossicle chain to the inner ear.
- It protects the auditory apparatus from intense vibrations.

- It equalizes the air pressure on both sides of the tympanic membrane to prevent it from rupturing.

The middle ear contains three small bones of the auditory ossicles: the malleus, or hammer; the incus, or anvil; and the stapes, or stirrup. These bones are linked like a chain and vibrate in place. The long process of the malleus fits into the incus, forming a true joint, and allows the two structures to move as a single unit. The proximal end of the stapes fits into the oval window, an opening that joins the middle and inner ear.

The eustachian tube connects the middle ear with the nasopharynx, equalizing air pressure on either side of the tympanic membrane. This tube also connects the ear's sterile area to the nasopharynx.

A normally functioning eustachian tube keeps the middle ear free from contaminants from the nasopharynx. Upper respiratory tract infections can affect the tube by obstructing middle ear drainage and causing otitis media or effusion.

Inner ear

The inner ear consists of closed, fluid-filled spaces within the temporal bone. It contains the bony labyrinth, which includes three connected structures: the vestibule, the semicircular canals, and the cochlea. These structures are lined with the membranous labyrinth. The fluid perilymph fills the space between the bony labyrinth and the membranous labyrinth.

The vestibule and semicircular canals help maintain equilibrium. The cochlea, a spiral chamber that resembles a snail shell, is the organ of hearing. The organ of Corti, part of the membranous labyrinth, contains hair cells that receive auditory sensations.

When sound waves reach the external ear, structures there transmit the waves through the auditory canal to the tympanic membrane, where they cause a chain reaction among the structures of the middle and inner ear. Finally, the cochlear branch of the acoustic nerve (cranial nerve VIII) transmits the vibrations to the temporal lobe of the cerebral cortex, where the brain interprets the sound.

Besides controlling hearing, structures in the middle and inner ear control balance. The semicircular canals of the inner ear contain cristae—hairlike structures that respond to body movements. Endolymph fluid bathes the cristae.

When a person moves, the cristae bend, releasing impulses through the vestibular portion of the acoustic nerve to the brain, which controls balance. When a person is stationary, nerve impulses to the brain orient him to this position, and the pressure of gravity on the inner ear helps him maintain balance.

Physical assessment

A complete eye assessment involves inspecting the external eye and lids, testing visual acuity, assessing eye muscle function, palpating the nasolacrimal sac, and examining intraocular structures with an ophthalmoscope. Examining the ears involves inspection, examination with an otoscope, and palpation.

Before starting your examination, gather the necessary equipment, including a good light source, one or two opaque cards, an ophthalmoscope, vision-test cards, gloves, tissues, and cotton-tipped applicators. For the ears you'll need an otoscope and a tuning fork. (See *Eyes and ears: Normal findings,* pages 212 and 213.)

EXAMINING THE EYES

Make sure your patient is seated comfortably and that you're seated at eye level with him.

INSPECTING THE EYES

Start your assessment by observing the patient's face. With the scalp line as the starting point, check that his eyes are in a normal position. They should be about one-third of the way down the face and about one eye's width apart from each other. Next assess the conjunctiva, cornea, anterior chamber, iris, pupil, and eyelid.

Eyelids

Each upper eyelid should cover the top quarter of the iris so the eyes look alike. Check for an excessive amount of visible sclera above the limbus (corneo-scleral junction). Ask the patient to open and close his eyes to see if they close completely. If the downward movement of the upper eyelid in down gaze is delayed, then the patient has lid lag, which is a common sign of hyperthyroidism.

Protrusion of the eyeball, called *exophthalmos* or *proptosis,* is common in patients with hyperthyroidism. It may also be seen with tumors, trauma, or inflammatory conditions. Assess the lids for redness, edema, inflammation, or lesions. Check for a stye, or hordeolum, a common eyelid lesion.

Also, inspect the eyes for excessive tearing or dryness. The eyelid margins should be pink, and the eyelashes should turn outward. Observe whether the lower eyelids turn inward toward the eyeball, called *entropion,* or outward, called *ectropion.* Examine the eyelids for lumps.

Before palpating the nasolacrimal sac, explain the procedure to the patient. Then put on gloves. With the patient's eyes closed, gently palpate the area below the inner canthus, noting tenderness, swelling, or discharge through the lacrimal point, which could indicate blockage of the nasolacrimal duct.

Conjunctiva

Next, have your patient look up. Gently pull the lower eyelid down to inspect the bulbar conjunctiva, the delicate mucous membrane that covers the exposed surface of the sclera. It should be clear and shiny. Note excessive redness or exudate. The palpebral conjunctiva in patients with a history of allergies may have a cobblestone appearance.

To examine the palpebral conjunctiva—the membrane that lines the eyelids—have the patient look down. Then lift the upper lid, holding the upper lashes against the eyebrow with your finger. The palpebral conjunctiva should be uniformly pink.

With the lid still secured, inspect the bulbar conjunctiva for color changes, foreign bodies, and edema. Also, observe the sclera's color, which should be white to buff. In black patients, you may see flecks of tan. A bluish discoloration may indicate scleral thinning.

Cornea

Examine the cornea by shining a penlight first from both sides and then from straight ahead. The cornea should be clear and without lesions. Test corneal sensitivity by lightly touching the cornea with a wisp of cotton. The patient should blink. If he doesn't, he may have suffered damage to the sensory fibers of cranial nerve V or to the motor fibers controlled by cranial nerve VI.

Keep in mind that people who wear contact lenses may have reduced sensitivity because they're accustomed to having foreign objects in their eyes.

Anterior chamber and iris

The anterior chamber of the eye is bordered anteriorly by the cornea and

Eyes and ears: Normal findings

Inspection

❑ No edema, scaling, or lesions on eyelids are apparent.

❑ Eyelids completely cover the corneas when closed.

❑ Eyelid color is the same as surrounding skin color.

❑ Palpebral fissures are of equal height.

❑ Margin of the upper lid falls between superior pupil margin and superior limbus.

❑ Upper eyelids are symmetrical and lesion free, and don't sag or droop when the patient opens his eyes.

❑ Eyelashes are evenly distributed and curve outward.

❑ Globe of the eye neither protrudes from nor is sunken into the orbit.

❑ Eyebrows are of equal size, color, and distribution.

❑ Nystagmus isn't present.

❑ Conjunctiva is clear with visible small blood vessels and no signs of drainage.

❑ White sclera is visible through conjunctiva.

❑ Anterior chamber is transparent and contains no visible material when you shine a penlight into the side of the eye.

❑ Cornea is transparent, smooth, and bright, with no visible irregularities or lesions.

❑ Lids of both eyes close when you stroke each cornea with a wisp of cotton, a test of cranial nerve V, the trigeminal nerve.

❑ Pupils are round and equal sized, and they react normally to light and accommodation.

❑ Both pupils constrict when you shine a light on one.

❑ Lacrimal structures are free from exudate, swelling, and excessive tearing.

❑ Eyes are properly aligned.

❑ Eye movement in each of the six cardinal fields of gaze is parallel.

❑ Auricles are bilaterally symmetrical and proportionately sized, with a vertical measurement of 1½" to 4" (3.5 to 10 cm).

❑ Tip of the ear crosses the eye-occiput line, an imaginary line extending from the lateral aspect of the eye to the occipital protuberance.

❑ Long axis of the ear is perpendicular to—or no more than 10 degrees from perpendicular to—the eye-occiput line.

❑ Ears and facial skin are the same color.

❑ No inflammation, lesions, or nodules are apparent.

❑ No cracking, thickening, scaling, or lesions are detectable behind the ear when you bend the auricle forward.

❑ There's no visible discharge from the auditory canal.

❑ External meatus is patent.

❑ Skin color on the mastoid process matches the skin color of the surrounding area.

❑ No redness or swelling is apparent.

❑ Otoscopic examination reveals normal drum landmarks and bright reflex, with no canal inflammation, bulging of membrane, or drainage.

Palpation

❑ Eyelids show no evidence of swelling or tenderness.

❑ Globes feel equally firm, not overly hard or spongy.

Eyes and ears: Normal findings (continued)

❑ Lacrimal sacs don't regurgitate fluid.
❑ No masses or tenderness on the auricle or tragus is detectable during manipulation.
❑ Lymph nodes are either small and nonpalpable and located behind the

auricle or discrete and mobile and have no signs of tenderness.
❑ Mastoid process has well-defined, bony edges, with no signs of tenderness.

---

posteriorly by the iris. The iris should appear flat, and the cornea should appear convex. Excess pressure in the eye—such as that caused by acute angle-closure glaucoma—may push the iris forward, making the anterior chamber appear very small. The irises should be the same size, color, and shape.

Pupils

The pupils should be equal in size, round, and about one-fourth the size of the irises in normal room light. About one person in four has asymmetrical pupils without disease. Unequal pupils generally indicate neurologic damage, iritis, glaucoma, or use of certain drugs. A fixed pupil that doesn't react to light can be an ominous neurologic sign.

Test the pupils for direct and consensual response. In a slightly darkened room, hold a penlight about 20″ (51 cm) from the patient's eyes, and direct the light at the eye from the side. Note the reaction of the pupil you're testing (direct response) and the opposite pupil (consensual response). They should both react the same way. Also, note sluggishness or inequality in the response. Repeat the test with the other pupil. *Note:* If you shine the light in a blind eye, neither pupil will respond. If

you shine the light in a seeing eye, both pupils will respond consensually.

To test the pupils for accommodation, place your finger about 4″ (10 cm) from the bridge of the patient's nose. Ask the patient to look at a fixed object in the distance and then to look at your finger. His pupils should constrict and his eyes converge as he focuses on your finger.

TESTING VISUAL ACUITY

To test your patient's far, near, and peripheral vision, use a Snellen chart and a near-vision chart. Before each test, ask the patient to remove corrective lenses, if he wears them.

Snellen chart

Have the patient sit or stand 20′ (6.1 m) from the chart, and then cover his left eye with an opaque object. Ask him to read the letters on one line of the chart and then to move his gaze downward to increasingly smaller lines until he can no longer discern all of the letters. Have him repeat the test covering his right eye.

Use the Snellen E chart to test visual acuity in young children and other patients who can't read. Cover the patient's left eye to check the right eye, point to an E on the chart, and ask the patient to point which way the letter

Visual acuity charts

The most commonly used charts for testing vision are the Snellen alphabet chart (left) and the Snellen E chart (right), the latter of which is used for young children and adults who can't read. Both charts are used to test distance vision and measure visual acuity. The patient reads each chart at a distance of 20' (6.1 m).

Recording results

Visual acuity is recorded as a fraction. The top number (20) is the distance between the patient and the chart. The bottom number is the distance from which a person with normal vision could read the line. The larger the bottom number, the poorer the patient's vision.

Age differences

In adults and children age 6 and older, normal vision is measured as 20/20. For children younger than age 6, normal vision varies. For children age 3 and younger, normal vision is 20/50; for children age 4, 20/40; and for children age 5, 20/30.

Snellen alphabet chart

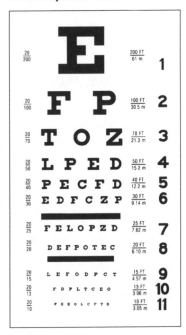

Snellen E chart

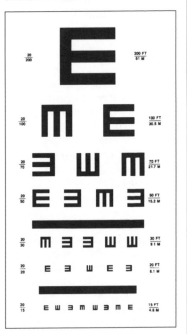

faces. Repeat the test with the left eye. (See *Visual acuity charts*.)

If the patient wears corrective lenses, have him repeat the test wearing them. If the test values between the two eyes differ by two lines, such as 20/30 in one eye and 20/50 in the other, suspect an abnormality such as amblyopia, especially in children. Record the vision with and without correction.

Near-vision chart

To test near vision, cover one of the patient's eyes with an opaque object, and hold a Rosenbaum near-vision card 14" (35.6 cm) from his eyes. Have him read the line with the smallest letters he can distinguish. Repeat the test with the other eye. If the patient wears corrective lenses, have him repeat the test while wearing them. Record the visual accommodation with and without lenses.

ASSESSING EYE MUSCLE FUNCTION

A thorough assessment of the eyes includes an evaluation of the extraocular muscles. To evaluate these muscles, you'll need to assess the corneal light reflex and the cardinal positions of gaze.

Corneal light reflex

To assess the corneal light reflex, ask the patient to look straight ahead; then shine a penlight on the bridge of his nose from 12" to 15" (30 to 38 cm) away. The light should fall at the same spot on each cornea. If it doesn't, the eyes aren't being held in the same plane by the extraocular muscles. This finding is common in patients with lack of muscle coordination, or strabismus.

Cardinal positions of gaze

Cardinal positions of gaze evaluates the oculomotor, trigeminal, and abducent nerves as well as the extraocular muscles. To perform this test, ask the pa-

tient to remain still while you hold a pencil or other small object directly in front of his nose at a distance of about 18" (46 cm).

Ask him to follow the object with his eyes, without moving his head. Then move the object to each of the six cardinal positions, returning to the midpoint after each movement. The six cardinal positions are right superior, right lateral, right inferior, left superior, left lateral, and left inferior. The patient's eyes should remain parallel as they move. Note abnormal findings such as nystagmus and diplopia, the failure of one eye to follow an object.

Cover-uncover test

The third test to assess extraocular muscle function is the cover-uncover test. This test usually isn't done unless you detect an abnormality during one of the two previous tests. To perform a cover-uncover test, have the patient stare at a wall on the other side of the room. Cover one eye and watch for movement in the uncovered eye. Remove the eye cover, and watch for movement again. Repeat the test with the other eye.

Eye movement while covering or uncovering the eye is considered abnormal. It may result from weak or paralyzed extraocular muscles, which may be caused by cranial nerve impairment.

EXAMINING INTRAOCULAR STRUCTURES

The ophthalmoscope allows you to directly observe internal structures of the eye. To see those structures properly, you'll need to adjust the lens disc. Use the black, plus numbers on the disc to focus on near objects such as the patient's cornea and lens. Use the red, minus numbers to focus on distant objects such as the retina.

Before the examination, have the patient remove contact lenses (if they're tinted) or eyeglasses, and darken the room to dilate his pupils and make your examination easier. Ask the patient to focus on a point behind you. Tell him that you'll be moving into his visual field and blocking his view. Also, explain that you'll be shining a bright light into his eye, which may be uncomfortable but not harmful. You should stand in front of the patient. Use your left eye to examine his left eye, and your right eye to examine his right eye.

Set the lens disc at zero, hold the ophthalmoscope about 4″ (10 cm) from the patient's eye, and direct the light through the pupil to elicit the red reflex, a reflection of light off the choroid. Check the red reflex for depth of color.

Now, move the ophthalmoscope closer to the eye. Adjust the lens disc so you can focus on the anterior chamber and lens. Look for clouding, foreign matter, or opacities. If the lens is opaque, indicating cataracts, you may not be able to complete the examination.

To examine the retina, start with the dial turned to zero. Rotate the lens-power disc to adjust for your refractive correction and the patient's refractive error. Now, observe the vitreous body for clarity. The first retinal structures you'll see are the blood vessels. Rotating the dial into the negative numbers will bring the blood vessels into focus. The arteries will look thinner and brighter than the veins.

Follow one of the vessels along its path toward the nose until you reach the optic disc, where all vessels in the eye originate. Examine arteriovenous crossings for arteriovenous nicking, or localized constriction of the vessels, which might be a sign of hypertension.

The optic disc is a creamy pink to yellow-orange structure with clear borders and a round-to-oval shape. With practice, you'll be able to identify the physiologic cup, a small depression that occupies about one-third of the disc's diameter. The disc may fill or exceed your field of vision. If you don't see it, follow a blood vessel toward the center until you do. The nasal border of the disc may be somewhat blurred.

Completely scan the retina by following four blood vessels from the optic disc to different peripheral areas. The retina should have a uniform color and be free from scars and pigmentation. As you scan, note lesions or hemorrhages. (See *Structures of the retina*.)

Finally, move the light laterally from the optic disc to locate the macula, the part of the eye most sensitive to light. It appears as a darker structure, free from blood vessels. Your view may be fleeting because most patients can't tolerate having a beam of light fall on the macula. If you locate it, ask the patient to gaze into the light.

EXAMINING THE EARS

To assess your patient's ears, you'll need to inspect and palpate the external structures, perform an otoscopic examination of the ear canal, and test hearing acuity.

External observations

Begin by observing the ears for position and symmetry. The top of the ear should line up with the outer corner of the eye, and the ears should look sym-

Structures of the retina

This illustration shows the complex anatomy of the retina and its structures.

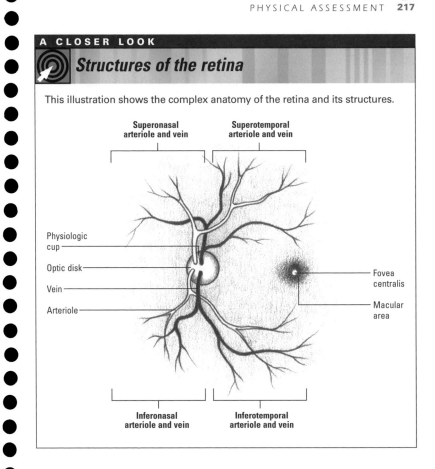

Superonasal
arteriole and vein

Superotemporal
arteriole and vein

Physiologic
cup

Optic disk

Vein

Arteriole

Fovea
centralis

Macular
area

Inferonasal
arteriole and vein

Inferotemporal
arteriole and vein

metrical, with an angle of attachment no more than 10 degrees. The face and ears should have the same shade and color.

Auricles that protrude from the head, or "lop" ears, are fairly common and don't affect hearing ability. However, low-set ears commonly accompany congenital disorders, including kidney problems.

Inspect the auricle for lesions, drainage, nodules, or redness. Pull the helix back, and note if it's tender. If pulling the ear back hurts the patient, he may have otitis externa.

Then inspect and palpate the mastoid area behind each auricle, noting tenderness, redness, or warmth. Finally, inspect the opening of the ear canal, noting discharge, redness, or odor. Patients normally have varying amounts of hair and cerumen in the ear canal.

Otoscopic examination

The next part of your ear assessment involves examining the patient's auditory canal, tympanic membrane, and

Using an otoscope

The otoscope is a useful tool for examining ears. For the best results, follow the tips below.

Inserting the speculum
Before inserting the speculum into the patient's ear, straighten the ear canal by grasping the auricle and pulling it up and back, as shown.

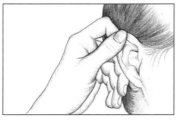

Positioning the scope
To examine the ear's external canal, hold the otoscope with the handle parallel to the patient's head, as shown. Bracing your hand firmly against his head keeps you from hitting the canal with the speculum.

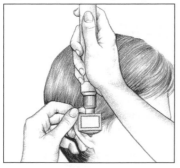

Viewing the structures
When the otoscope is positioned properly, you should see the tympanic membrane structures shown here.

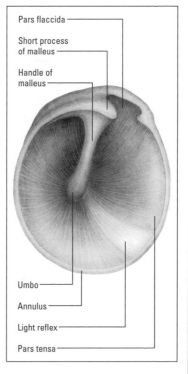

Pars flaccida

Short process of malleus

Handle of malleus

Umbo

Annulus

Light reflex

Pars tensa

malleus with the otoscope. Before inserting the speculum into the patient's ear canal, check the canal for foreign particles or discharge. (See *Using an otoscope.*)

Then palpate the tragus—the cartilaginous projection anterior to the external opening of the ear—and pull the auricle up. If this area is tender, don't insert the speculum. The patient could have otitis externa, and inserting the speculum could be painful.

To insert the speculum of the otoscope, tilt the patient's head away from you. Then grasp the superior posterior auricle with your thumb and index finger and pull it up and back to straighten the canal. Because everyone's ear canal is shaped differently, vary the angle of the speculum until you can see the tympanic membrane. If your patient is younger than age 3, pull the auricle down and out to get a good view of the membrane.

Insert the speculum to about one-third its length when inspecting the canal. Be sure to insert it gently because the inner two-thirds of the canal is sensitive to pressure. Note the color of the cerumen. Cerumen that's grayish brown and dry-looking is old. The elderly patient may have harder, drier cerumen because of rigid cilia in the ear canal. The external canal should be free from inflammation and scaling.

If excessive cerumen obstructs your view of the tympanic membrane, don't try to remove it with an instrument because you could cause the patient excessive pain. Instead, use ceruminolytic drops and warm water irrigation, as ordered. If the tympanic membrane has perforated, the cerumen should be removed by a physician or other qualified provider.

You may need to carefully rotate the speculum for a complete view of the tympanic membrane. The membrane should be pearl gray, glistening, and transparent. The annulus should be white and denser than the rest of the membrane. Inspect the membrane carefully for bulging, retraction, bleeding, lesions, or perforations, especially at the periphery. If the patient is elderly, the eardrum may appear cloudy.

Now, examine the membrane for the light reflex. The light reflex in the right ear should be between 4 and 6 o'clock; in the left ear, between 6 and 8 o'clock. If the reflex is displaced or absent, the patient's tympanic membrane may be bulging, inflamed, or retracted.

Finally, look for the bony landmarks. The malleus will appear as a dense, white streak at the 12 o'clock position. At the top of the light reflex, you'll find the umbo, the inferior point of the malleus.

Hearing acuity tests

The last part of an ear assessment is testing the patient's hearing, using Weber's and Rinne tests. These tests assess conductive hearing loss, impaired sound transmission to the inner ear, sensorineural hearing loss, impaired auditory nerve conduction, and inner ear function.

Weber's test is performed when the patient reports diminished or lost hearing in one ear. This test uses a tuning fork to evaluate bone conduction. The tuning fork should be tuned to the frequency of normal human speech, 512 cycles/second.

To perform Weber's test, strike the tuning fork lightly against your hand, and then place the fork on the patient's forehead at the midline or on top of his head. If he hears the tone equally well in both ears, record this result as normal. If he hears the tone better in one ear, record the result as right or left lateralization.

Positioning the tuning fork

Whether you're using Weber's test or the Rinne test to assess a patient's hearing, proper positioning of the tuning fork is key to achieving accurate test results.

Weber's test
With the tuning fork vibrating lightly, position the tip on the patient's forehead at the midline, as shown. Or place the tuning fork on the top of the patient's head.

Rinne test
Strike the tuning fork against your hand, and then hold it behind the patient's ear, as shown. When the patient tells you the tone has stopped, move the still-vibrating tuning fork to the opening of her ear.

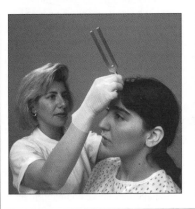
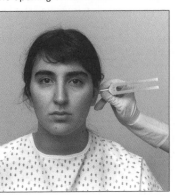

During lateralization, the tone sounds louder in the ear with hearing loss because bone conducts the tone to the ear. Because the unaffected ear picks up other sounds, it doesn't hear the tone as clearly.

Perform the Rinne test after Weber's test, to compare air conduction of sound with bone conduction of sound. To perform this test, strike the tuning fork against your hand, and then place it over the patient's mastoid process. Ask the patient to tell you when the tone stops, and note this time in seconds. Next, move the still-vibrating

tuning fork to the opening of the ear without touching the ear. Ask the patient to tell you when the tone stops. Note the time in seconds. (See *Positioning the tuning fork*.)

The patient should hear the air-conducted tone twice as long as she hears the bone-conducted tone. If she doesn't hear the air-conducted tone longer than the bone-conducted tone, she has a conductive hearing loss in the affected ear.

Guidelines for a 3-minute assessment

When your patient has a problem related to the eyes or ears, perform your 3-minute assessment as described below. Such assessment includes making general observations, checking the patient's vital signs, and focusing on the patient's chief sign or symptom.

MAKING GENERAL OBSERVATIONS

Begin your assessment by looking at the overall appearance of the eyes, including the eyebrows, eyelids, eyelashes, and eyeballs. Note asymmetry or gross abnormalities, such as ptosis. Look for redness, crusting, or excessive tearing. Observe whether the patient wears contact lenses or glasses. Then look at the skin color around his eyes and compare it with the rest of his facial skin, noting signs of trauma.

Look at both ears for symmetry, shape, contour, and color. Look for any obvious lesions, drainage, or swelling. Look for hearing aids. Listen to your patient's tone of voice and note irregularities such as excessive loudness.

CHECKING VITAL SIGNS

Check the patient's vital signs, particularly his temperature, a key indicator of ear infection. Changes in pulse rate and blood pressure may result from head injuries, which can cause eye and ear problems for the patient.

FOCUSING ON THE CHIEF SIGN OR SYMPTOM

After you've made general observations and checked the patient's vital signs, you'll want to focus on the patient's chief eye or ear sign or symptom for the history and physical assessment.

Further assessment

You may need to perform a complete neurologic examination in addition to assessing the eyes and ears. After obtaining a history and performing the physical assessment, you'll begin to form a diagnostic impression. (See *Eyes and ears: Interpreting your findings,* pages 222 and 223.)

Common signs and symptoms

A patient may seek care for any of a number of signs and symptoms related to the eyes and ears. Some common ones are earache, eye discharge, hearing loss, and visual blurring.

EARACHES

Earaches usually result from disorders of the external and middle ear associated with infection, obstruction, or trauma. Their severity ranges from a feeling of fullness or blockage to deep, boring pain; at times, they may be diffi-

(Text continues on page 224.)

DIAGNOSTIC IMPRESSION

➡ *Eyes and ears: Interpreting your findings*

After you assess the patient, a group of findings may lead you to suspect a particular disorder. The chart below shows common groups of findings for the signs and symptoms of the eyes and ears, along with their probable causes.

Sign or symptom and findings	Probable cause
Earache	
• Sensation of blockage or fullness in the ear • Itching • Partial hearing loss • Possibly dizziness	Cerumen impaction
• Mild to moderate ear pain that occurs with tragus manipulation • Low-grade fever • Sticky yellow or purulent ear discharge • Partial hearing loss • Feeling of blockage in the ear • Swelling of the tragus, external meatus, and external canal • Lymphadenopathy	Otitis externa, acute
• Severe, deep, throbbing ear pain • Hearing loss • High fever • Bulging, fiery red eardrum	Otitis media, acute suppurative
Eye discharge	
• Purulent or mucopurulent, greenish-white discharge that occurs unilaterally • Sticky crusts that form on the eyelids during sleep • Itching and burning • Excessive tearing • Sensation of a foreign body in the eye	Bacterial conjunctivitis
• Scant but continuous purulent discharge that's easily expressed from the tear sac • Excessive tearing • Pain and tenderness near the tear sac • Eyelid inflammation and edema noticeable around the lacrimal punctum	Dacryocystitis

Eyes and ears: Interpreting your findings (continued)

Sign or symptom and findings	Probable cause
Eye discharge (continued)	
• Continuous frothy discharge • Chronically red eyes with inflamed lid margins • Soft, foul-smelling, cheesy yellow discharge elicited by pressure on the meibomian glands	Meibomianitis
Hearing loss	
• Conductive hearing loss • Ear pain or a feeling of fullness • Nasal congestion • Conjunctivitis	Allergies
• Sudden or intermittent conductive hearing loss • Bony projections visible in the ear canal • Normal tympanic membrane	Osteoma
• Abrupt hearing loss • Ear pain • Tinnitus • Vertigo • Sense of fullness in the ear	Tympanic membrane perforation
Visual blurring	
• Gradual visual blurring • Halo vision • Visual glare in bright light • Progressive vision loss • Gray pupil that later turns milky white	Cataract
• Constant morning headache that decreases in severity during the day • Possible severe, throbbing headache • Restlessness • Confusion • Nausea and vomiting • Seizures • Decreased level of consciousness	Hypertension
• Paroxysmal attacks of severe, throbbing, unilateral or bilateral headache • Nausea and vomiting • Sensitivity to light and noise • Sensory or visual auras	Migraine headache

cult to localize precisely. This common symptom may be intermittent or continuous and may develop suddenly or gradually.

History

Ask the patient to characterize the earache. How long has he had it? Is it intermittent or continuous? Is it painful or slightly annoying? Can he localize the site of ear pain? Does he have pain in other areas such as the jaw?

Ask about recent ear injury or other trauma. Does swimming or showering trigger ear discomfort? Is discomfort associated with itching? If so, find out where the itching is most intense and when it began. Ask about ear drainage and, if present, have the patient characterize it. Does he hear ringing or noise in his ears? Ask about dizziness or vertigo. Does the vertigo worsen when the patient changes position? Does he have difficulty swallowing, hoarseness, neck pain, or pain when he opens his mouth?

Find out if the patient has recently had a head cold or problems with his eyes, mouth, teeth, jaws, sinuses, or throat. Disorders in these areas may refer pain to the ear along the cranial nerves.

Physical assessment

Begin your physical examination by inspecting the external ear for redness, drainage, swelling, or deformity. Then apply pressure to the mastoid process and tragus to elicit any tenderness. Using an otoscope, examine the external auditory canal for lesions, bleeding, discharge, impacted cerumen, foreign bodies, tenderness, or swelling. Examine the tympanic membrane: Is it intact? Is it the normal pearly gray? Look for tympanic membrane landmarks: the cone of light, umbo, pars tensa, and the handle and short process of the malleus. Perform the watch tick, whispered voice, Rinne, and Weber's tests to assess the patient for hearing loss.

Analysis

The particular symptoms your patient describes and the signs you observe help pinpoint the cause. Pain caused by touching or pulling the ear, for instance, usually indicates an external ear infection; a deep throbbing pain, a middle ear disorder. A severely inflamed outer ear may result from a swollen or completely blocked ear canal. A feeling of pressure or blockage can stem from a eustachian tube dysfunction that creates negative pressure in the middle ear or from muscle spasm or temporomandibular joint arthralgia.

PEDIATRIC TIP

Common causes of earache in children are acute otitis media and insertion of foreign bodies that become lodged or infected. Be alert for crying or ear tugging in a young child—nonverbal clues to earache.

To examine the child's ears, place him in a supine position with his arms extended and held securely by his parent. Then hold the otoscope with the handle pointing toward the top of the child's head, and brace it against him using one or two fingers. Because an ear examination may upset the child with an earache, save it for the end of your physical examination.

EYE DISCHARGE

Usually associated with conjunctivitis, an eye discharge is the excretion of any substance other than tears. This common sign may occur in one or both eyes, producing scant to copious discharge. The discharge may be purulent, frothy, mucoid, cheesy, serous, clear, or stringy and white. Sometimes, the discharge can be expressed by applying pressure to the tear sac, punctum, meibomian glands, or canaliculus.

History
Begin your evaluation by finding out when the discharge began. Does it occur at certain times of day or in connection with certain activities? If the patient complains of pain, ask him to show you its exact location and to describe its character. Is the pain dull, continuous, sharp, or stabbing? Do his eyes itch or burn? Do they tear excessively? Are they sensitive to light? Does he feel like something is in them?

Physical assessment
After checking vital signs, carefully inspect the eye discharge. Note its amount and consistency. Then test visual acuity, with and without correction. Examine external eye structures, beginning with the unaffected eye to prevent cross-contamination. Check for eyelid edema, entropion, crusts, lesions, and trichiasis. Next, ask the patient to blink as you watch for impaired lid movement. If the eyes seem to bulge, measure them with an exophthalmometer. Test the six cardinal fields of gaze. Examine for conjunctival injection and follicles and for corneal cloudiness or white lesions.

Analysis
Eye discharge is common in patients with an inflammatory or infectious eye disorder, but it may also occur in patients with certain systemic disorders. Because this sign may accompany a disorder that threatens vision, it must be assessed and treated immediately.

PEDIATRIC TIP
In infants, the prophylactic eye medication silver nitrate commonly causes eye irritation and discharge. However, in children, discharges usually result from eye trauma, eye infection, or upper respiratory tract infection.

HEARING LOSS
Hearing loss affects nearly 16 million U.S. residents. It may be temporary or permanent, and partial or complete. This common symptom may involve reception of low-, middle-, or high-frequency tones. If the hearing loss doesn't affect speech frequencies, the patient may be unaware of it.

History
If the patient reports hearing loss, ask him to describe it fully. Is it unilateral or bilateral? Continuous or intermittent? Ask about a family history of hearing loss. Then obtain the patient's medical history, noting chronic ear infections, ear surgery, and ear or head trauma. Has the patient recently had an upper respiratory tract infection? After taking a drug history, have the patient describe his occupation and work environment.

Next, explore associated signs and symptoms. Does the patient have ear pain? If so, is it unilateral or bilateral? Continuous or intermittent? Ask the patient if he has noticed discharge from one or both ears. If so, have him describe its color and consistency, and note when it began. Does he hear ringing, buzzing, hissing, or other noises in one or both ears? If so, are the noises constant or intermittent? Does he experience dizziness? If so, when did he first notice it?

Physical assessment

Begin the physical examination by inspecting the external ear for inflammation, boils, foreign bodies, and discharge. Gently manipulate the auricle and note any discomfort. Then apply pressure to the tragus and mastoid to elicit tenderness. If you detect tenderness or external ear abnormalities, notify the physician to discuss whether an otoscopic examination should be done. During the otoscopic examination, note color change, perforation, bulging, or retraction of the tympanic membrane, which normally looks like a shiny, pearl gray cone.

Next, evaluate the patient's hearing acuity, using the ticking watch and whispered voice tests. Then perform Weber's and Rinne tests to obtain a preliminary evaluation of the type and degree of hearing loss.

Analysis

Normally, sound waves enter the external auditory canal, then travel to the middle ear's tympanic membrane and ossicles—that is, the incus, malleus, and stapes—and into the inner ear's cochlea. The cochlear division of the eighth cranial, or auditory, nerve carries the sound impulse to the brain. This type of sound transmission, air conduction, is normally better than bone conduction—sound transmission through bone to the inner ear.

Hearing loss can be classified as conductive, sensorineural, mixed, and functional. Conductive hearing loss results from external or middle ear disorders that block sound transmission. This type of hearing loss usually responds to medical or surgical intervention, or in some cases, both. Sensorineural hearing loss results from disorders of the inner ear or of the eighth cranial nerve. Mixed hearing loss combines aspects of conductive and sensorineural hearing loss. Functional hearing loss results from psychological factors rather than identifiable organic damage.

Hearing loss may also result from trauma, infection, allergy, a tumor, certain systemic and hereditary disorders, or the use of ototoxic drugs and treatments. In most cases, though, it results from presbycusis, a sensorineural hearing loss that usually affects people older than age 50. Other physiologic causes of hearing loss include cerumen impaction; barotitis media, or unequal pressure on the eardrum, associated with descent in an airplane or elevator, diving, or close proximity to an explosion; and chronic exposure to noise over 90 decibels, which can occur on the job, with certain hobbies, or from listening to live or recorded music.

PEDIATRIC TIP

About 3,000 profoundly deaf infants are born in the United States each year. In about half of these infants, hereditary disorders (such as Paget's disease, and Alport's, Hurler's, and Klippel-Feil syndromes) cause the typically sensorineural hearing loss. Nonhereditary disorders associated with congenital sensorineural hearing loss include Usher's syndrome, albinism, onychodystrophy, cochlear dysplasias, and Pendred's, Waardenburg's, and Jervell and Lange-Nielsen syndromes. This type of hearing loss may also result from maternal use of ototoxic drugs, birth trauma, and anoxia during or after birth.

Mumps is the most common pediatric cause of unilateral sensorineural hearing loss. Other causes are meningitis, measles, influenza, and acute febrile illness. Disorders that may produce congenital conductive hearing loss include atresia, ossicle malformation, and other abnormalities. Serous otitis media commonly causes bilateral conductive hearing loss in children. Conductive hearing loss may also occur in children who put foreign objects in their ears.

Hearing disorders in children may lead to speech, language, and learning problems. Early identification and treatment of hearing loss is thus crucial to avoid incorrectly labeling the child as mentally retarded, brain damaged, or slow.

When assessing an infant or a young child for hearing loss, remember that you can't use a tuning fork. Instead, test the startle reflex in infants younger than age 6 months, or have an audiologist test brain stem evoked response in neonates, infants, and young children. Also, obtain a gestational, perinatal, and family history from the parents.

GERIATRIC TIP
In older patients, presbycusis, the loss of the ability to discriminate sounds, may be aggravated by exposure to noise as well as other factors.

VISUAL BLURRING
Visual blurring is a common symptom that refers to the loss of visual acuity with indistinct visual details.

History
If the patient isn't in distress, ask him how long he has had the visual blurring. Does it occur only at certain times? Ask about associated symptoms, such as pain or discharge. If visual blurring followed injury, obtain details of the accident, and ask if vision was impaired immediately after the injury. Obtain a medical and drug history.

Physical assessment
Inspect the patient's eye, noting lid edema, drainage, or conjunctival or scleral redness. Also note an irregularly shaped iris, which may indicate previous trauma, and excessive blinking, which may indicate corneal damage. Check for pupillary changes, and test visual acuity in both eyes. If the patient has visual blurring accompanied by sudden, severe eye pain, a history of trauma, or sudden vision loss, perform an ophthalmologic examination. If the patient has a penetrating or perforating eye injury, don't touch the eye.

Analysis
Visual blurring may result from an eye injury, a neurologic or eye disorder, or a disorder with vascular complications, such as diabetes mellitus. Visual blurring may also result from mucus passing over the cornea, refractive errors, improperly fitted contact lenses, or the use of certain drugs.

PEDIATRIC TIP
Visual blurring in children may stem from congenital syphilis, congenital cataracts, refractive errors, an eye injury or infection, or increased intracranial pressure. Refer the child to an ophthalmologist if appropriate.

Test vision in school-age children as you would in adults; test children ages 3 to 6 with the Snellen symbol chart. Test toddlers with Allen cards, each illustrated with a familiar object such as an animal. Ask the child to cover one eye and identify the objects as you flash them. Then, ask him to identify them as you gradually back away. Record the maximum distance at which he can identify at least three pictures.

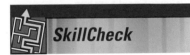

SkillCheck

1. Disorders in which parts of the ear usually result in earaches?
  a. Inner and middle ear
  b. Inner and external ear
  c. Middle and external ear
  d. Tragus and eardrum
Answer: c. Disorders of the middle and external ear that are associated with infection, obstruction, or trauma usually result in an earache.

2. Eye discharge is usually associated with:
  a. hypertension.
  b. conjunctivitis.
  c. otitis externa.
  d. meibomianitis.
Answer: b. Eye discharge is a common symptom usually associated with conjunctivitis, which can be allergic, bacterial, viral, or fungal.

3. Which type of hearing loss results from disorders of the inner ear or of the eighth cranial nerve?
  a. Conductive hearing loss
  b. Sensorineural hearing loss
  c. Mixed hearing loss
  d. Functional hearing loss
Answer: b. Sensorineural hearing loss results from disorders of the inner ear or the eighth cranial nerve. Conductive hearing loss results from external or middle ear disorders that block sound transmission; mixed hearing loss, from a combination of conductive and sensorineural problems; and functional hearing loss, from psychological factors.

4. Which item is used to test for corneal sensitivity?
  a. Cotton-tipped applicator
  b. Gauze pad
  c. Tissue
  d. Wisp of cotton
Answer: d. A wisp of cotton is the only safe object to use, to avoid causing corneal abrasion or irritation.

5. What should you palpate before inserting the otoscope into your patient's ear?
  a. Tragus
  b. Lymph nodes
  c. Helix
  d. Earlobe
Answer: a. Palpate the tragus before inserting the otoscope. If the patient has a tender tragus, a sign of otitis externa, otoscopic examination could be painful.

Nose and throat

Smell and taste allow us to connect with the world around us and take pleasure in our surroundings. These senses, like seeing and hearing, play vital roles in daily life. Although problems related to the structures that make these senses possible are common, such problems should be thoroughly assessed.

Anatomy and physiology

To perform an accurate 3-minute assessment you need to understand the anatomy and physiology of the nose and throat.

NOSE

The nose is more than the sensory organ of smell. It also plays a key role in the respiratory system by filtering, warming, and humidifying inhaled air. When you assess the nose, you'll typically assess the paranasal sinuses as well.

The lower two-thirds of the external nose consists of flexible cartilage, and the upper one-third is rigid bone. Posteriorly, the internal nose merges with the pharynx. Anteriorly, it merges with the external nose.

The internal and external nose are divided vertically by the nasal septum, which is straight at birth and in early life but becomes slightly deviated or deformed in almost every adult. Only the posterior end, which separates the posterior nares, remains constantly in the midline.

Air entering the nose passes through the vestibule, which is lined with coarse hair that helps filter out dust. Olfactory receptors lie above the vestibule in the roof of the nasal cavity and the upper one-third of the septum. Known as the olfactory region, this area is rich in capillaries and mucus-producing goblet cells that help warm, moisten, and clean inhaled air. Kiesselbach's area, the most common site of nosebleeds, is located in the septum's anterior portion. Because of its rich blood supply, the nasal mucosa is redder in color than the oral mucosa.

Further along the nasal passage are the superior, middle, and inferior turbinates. Separated by grooves called meatus, the curved bony turbinates and their mucosal covering ease breathing by warming, filtering, and humidifying inhaled air.

Four pairs of paranasal sinuses open into the internal nose, including the:
- maxillary sinuses, located on the cheeks below the eyes
- frontal sinuses, located above the eyebrows

Structures of the nose and mouth

These illustrations show the anatomic structures of the nose, mouth, and oropharynx.

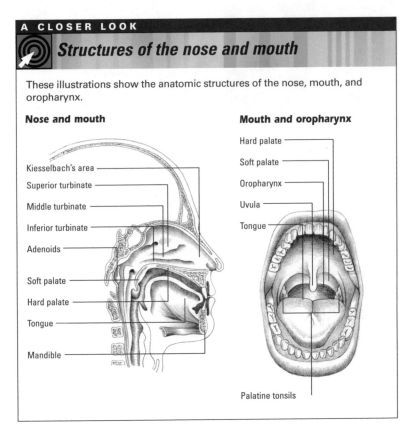

Nose and mouth

Kiesselbach's area
Superior turbinate
Middle turbinate
Inferior turbinate
Adenoids
Soft palate
Hard palate
Tongue
Mandible

Mouth and oropharynx

Hard palate
Soft palate
Oropharynx
Uvula
Tongue

Palatine tonsils

■ ethmoidal and sphenoidal sinuses, located behind the eyes and nose in the head.

The sinuses serve as resonators for sound production and provide mucus. Although you can assess the maxillary and frontal sinuses, the ethmoidal and sphenoidal sinuses aren't readily accessible. (See *Structures of the nose and mouth.*)

The small openings between the sinuses and the nasal cavity can easily become obstructed because they're lined with mucous membranes that can become inflamed and swollen.

THROAT

The throat, or pharynx, is divided into the nasopharynx, the oropharynx, and the laryngopharynx. Located within the throat are the hard and soft palates, the uvula, and the tonsils. The mucous membrane lining the throat normally is smooth and bright pink to light red.

The neck is formed by the cervical vertebrae and the major neck and shoulder muscles, together with their ligaments. Other important structures of the neck include the trachea, thyroid gland, and chains of lymph nodes.

The thyroid gland lies in the anterior neck, just below the larynx. Its two cone-shaped lobes are located on either side of the trachea and are connected by an isthmus below the cricoid cartilage, which gives the gland its butterfly shape. The largest endocrine gland, the thyroid produces the hormones triiodothyronine and thyroxine, which affect the metabolic reactions of every cell in the body.

Physical assessment

Examining the nose and throat mainly involves using inspection, palpation, and auscultation. An otoscope is needed for these assessments. (See *Nose and throat: Normal findings*, page 232.)

EXAMINING THE NOSE AND SINUSES

A complete examination of the nose also includes checking the sinuses. To perform this examination, use inspection and palpation.

Inspecting and palpating the nose

Begin by observing the patient's nose for position, symmetry, and color. Note variations, such as discoloration, swelling, or deformity. Variations in size and shape are largely due to differences in cartilage and in the amount of fibroadipose tissue.

Check for nasal discharge or flaring in infants. If discharge is present, note the color, quantity, and consistency. If you notice flaring, look for other signs of respiratory distress.

To test nasal patency and olfactory nerve (cranial nerve I) function, ask the patient to block one nostril and inhale a familiar aromatic substance through the other nostril. Possible substances include soap, coffee, citrus, tobacco, and nutmeg. Ask him to identify the aroma. Then repeat the process with the other nostril, using a different aroma.

Now, inspect the nasal cavity. Ask the patient to tilt his head back slightly, and then push the tip of his nose up. Use the light from the otoscope to illuminate the nasal cavities. Check for severe deviation or perforation of the nasal septum. Examine the vestibule and turbinates for redness, inflammation, softness, and discharge.

Examine the nostrils by direct inspection, using a nasal speculum and a penlight or small flashlight, or an otoscope with a short, wide-tip attachment. Have the patient sit in front of you with his head tilted back. Put on gloves, and insert the tip of the closed nasal speculum into one nostril to the point where the blade widens. Slowly open the speculum as wide as possible without causing discomfort. Shine the flashlight in the nostril to illuminate the area.

Observe the color and patency of the nostril, and check for exudate. The mucosa should be moist, pink to light red, and free from lesions and polyps. After inspecting one nostril, close the speculum, remove it, and inspect the other nostril.

Finally, palpate the patient's nose with your thumb and forefinger, checking for pain, tenderness, swelling, and deformity.

Nose and throat: Normal findings

Inspection
Nose
❑ Nose is symmetrical and lesion free, with no deviation of the septum or discharge.
❑ No nasal flaring is apparent.
❑ Frontal and maxillary sinuses are nonedematous.
❑ Patient can identify familiar odors.
❑ Nasal mucosa is pinkish red, with no visible lesions and no purulent drainage.
❑ There is no evidence of foreign bodies or dried blood in the nose.
Mouth
❑ Lips are pink, with no dryness, cracking, lesions, or cyanosis.
❑ Facial structures are symmetrical.
❑ Patient can purse his lips and puff out his cheeks, a sign of an adequately functioning cranial nerve VII (facial nerve).
❑ Patient can easily open and close his mouth.
❑ Oral mucosa is light pink and moist, with no ulcers or lesions.
❑ Palate is white and hard, or pink and soft.
❑ Gums are pink, with no tartar, inflammation, or hemorrhage.
❑ Teeth are intact, with no signs of occlusion, caries, or breakage.
❑ Tongue is pink, with no swelling, coating, ulcers, or lesions.
❑ Tongue moves easily and without tremor, a sign of a properly functioning cranial nerve XII (hypoglossal nerve).
❑ Anterior and posterior arches are free from swelling and inflammation.
❑ Posterior pharynx is free from lesions and inflammation.
❑ There is no unusual odor to the breath.

❑ Tonsils are lesion free and the right size for the patient's age.
❑ The uvula moves upward when the patient says "ah," and the gag reflex occurs when a tongue blade touches the posterior pharynx, both of which are signs of properly functioning cranial nerves IX and X.
Throat
❑ Neck is symmetrical with intact skin and no visible pulsations, masses, swelling, venous distention, or thyroid or lymph node enlargement.
❑ There is normal rising of the larynx, trachea, and thyroid as the patient swallows.

Palpation
Nose
❑ External nose is free from structural deviation, tenderness, and swelling.
❑ Frontal and maxillary sinuses are free from tenderness and edema.
Mouth
❑ Lips are free from pain and induration.
❑ No lesions, unusual color, tenderness, or swelling is apparent on the tongue's posterior and lateral surfaces.
❑ Floor of the mouth is free from tenderness, nodules, and swelling.
Throat
❑ Lymph nodes are nonpalpable or feel soft, mobile, and nontender.
❑ Thyroid isthmus rises when the patient swallows.

Auscultation
Throat
❑ No bruits are heard over the carotid arteries or over the thyroid gland.

Examining the sinuses

Next examine the frontal and maxillary sinuses. (Remember that the ethmoidal and sphenoidal sinuses are unpalpable.) If the frontal and maxillary sinuses are infected, you can assume that the other sinuses are as well.

Begin by checking for swelling around the eyes, especially over the sinus area. Then palpate the sinuses, checking for tenderness. (See *Palpating the maxillary sinuses*.) To palpate the frontal sinuses, place your thumbs above the patient's eyes just under the bony ridges of the upper orbits, and place your fingertips on his forehead. Apply gentle pressure. Next palpate the maxillary sinuses. If the patient complains of tenderness, use transillumination to see if the sinuses are filled with fluid or pus. Transillumination can also help reveal tumors and obstructions.

To transilluminate the sinuses, darken the room. Place a penlight on the supraorbital ring and direct the light upward to illuminate the frontal sinuses just above the eyebrow. Then place the penlight on the patient's cheekbone just below his eye and ask him to open his mouth. The light should transilluminate easily and equally.

EXAMINING THE MOUTH, THROAT, AND NECK

Assessing the mouth and throat requires inspection and palpation; assessing the neck, auscultation as well.

Assessing the mouth and throat

First, inspect the patient's lips. They should be pink, moist, symmetrical, and without lesions. A bluish hue or flecked pigmentation is common in dark-skinned patients. Put on gloves,

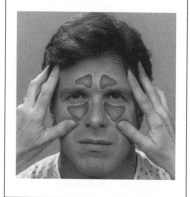

Palpating the maxillary sinuses

To palpate the maxillary sinuses, gently press your thumbs on each side of the nose just below the cheekbones, as shown. The illustration also shows the location of the frontal sinuses.

and palpate the lips for lumps or surface abnormalities.

Use a tongue blade and a bright light to inspect the oral mucosa. Have the patient open his mouth, and then place the tongue blade on top of his tongue. The oral mucosa should be pink, smooth, moist, and free from lesions and unusual odors. Increased pigmentation is seen in dark-skinned patients.

Next observe the gingivae: They should be pink and moist, have clearly defined margins at each tooth, and not be retracted. The gums of dark complexioned patients may have brown spots or patches. Inspect the teeth, noting their number, condition, and whether any are missing or crowded.

Finally, inspect the tongue. It should be midline, moist, pink, and free of lesions. The posterior surface should be smooth, and the anterior surface should be slightly rough with small fissures. The tongue should move easily in all directions, and it should lie straight to the front at rest.

Ask the patient to raise the tip of his tongue and touch his palate directly behind his front teeth. Inspect the ventral surface of the tongue and the floor of the mouth. Next, wrap a piece of gauze around the tip of the tongue and move the tongue first to one side then the other to inspect the lateral borders. They should be smooth and even-textured.

Inspect the patient's oropharynx by asking him to open his mouth while you shine the penlight on the uvula and palate. You may need to insert a tongue blade into the mouth and depress the tongue. Place the tongue blade slightly off center to avoid eliciting the gag reflex. The uvula and oropharynx should be pink and moist, without inflammation or exudate. The tonsils should be pink and not hypertrophied. Ask the patient to say "ah," and then observe for movement of the soft palate and uvula.

Finally, palpate the lips, tongue, and oropharynx. Note lumps, lesions, ulcers, or edema of the lips or tongue. Assess the patient's gag reflex by gently touching the back of the pharynx with a cotton-tipped applicator or tongue blade. This should produce a bilateral response.

Inspecting and palpating the neck

First, observe the patient's neck. It should be symmetrical and the skin should be intact. No visible pulsations, masses, swelling, venous distention, or thyroid or lymph node enlargement should be present. Ask the patient to move his head through the entire range of motion and to shrug his shoulders. Also ask him to swallow. Note rising of the larynx, trachea, and thyroid.

Palpate the patient's neck to gather more data. Using the finger pads of both hands, bilaterally palpate the chain of lymph nodes under the patient's chin in the preauricular area; then proceed to the area under and behind the ears. (See *Locating lymph nodes.*) Assess the nodes for size, shape, mobility, consistency, and tenderness, comparing nodes on one side with those on the other.

Then palpate the trachea, normally located midline in the neck. Place your thumbs along each side of the trachea near the lower part of the neck. Assess whether the distance between the trachea's outer edge and the sternocleidomastoid muscle is equal on both sides.

To palpate the thyroid, stand behind the patient and put your hands around his neck, with the fingers of both hands over the lower trachea. Ask him to swallow as you feel the thyroid isthmus. The isthmus should rise with swallowing because it lies across the trachea, just below the cricoid cartilage.

Displace the thyroid to the right and then to the left, palpating both lobes for enlargement, nodules, tenderness, or a gritty sensation. (See *The thyroid gland,* page 236.) Lowering the patient's chin slightly and turning toward the side you're palpating helps relax the muscle and may facilitate your assessment.

Auscultating the neck
Finally, auscultate the neck. Using light pressure on the bell of the stethoscope,

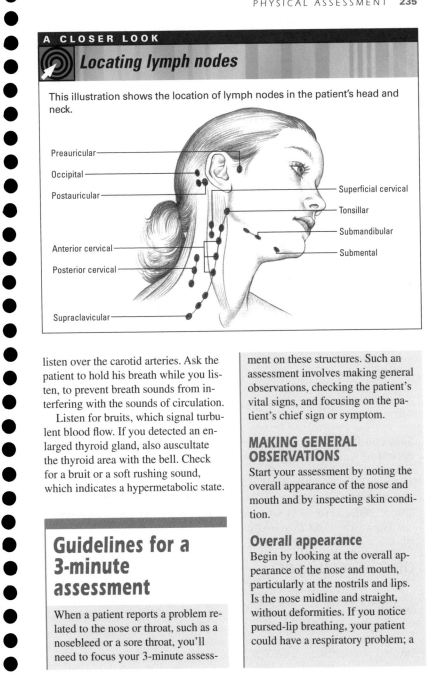

A CLOSER LOOK

Locating lymph nodes

This illustration shows the location of lymph nodes in the patient's head and neck.

Preauricular

Occipital

Postauricular

Anterior cervical

Posterior cervical

Supraclavicular

Superficial cervical

Tonsillar

Submandibular

Submental

listen over the carotid arteries. Ask the patient to hold his breath while you listen, to prevent breath sounds from interfering with the sounds of circulation.

Listen for bruits, which signal turbulent blood flow. If you detected an enlarged thyroid gland, also auscultate the thyroid area with the bell. Check for a bruit or a soft rushing sound, which indicates a hypermetabolic state.

Guidelines for a 3-minute assessment

When a patient reports a problem related to the nose or throat, such as a nosebleed or a sore throat, you'll need to focus your 3-minute assess-

ment on these structures. Such an assessment involves making general observations, checking the patient's vital signs, and focusing on the patient's chief sign or symptom.

MAKING GENERAL OBSERVATIONS

Start your assessment by noting the overall appearance of the nose and mouth and by inspecting skin condition.

Overall appearance

Begin by looking at the overall appearance of the nose and mouth, particularly at the nostrils and lips. Is the nose midline and straight, without deformities. If you notice pursed-lip breathing, your patient could have a respiratory problem; a

The thyroid gland

This illustration shows the structure and location of the thyroid gland.

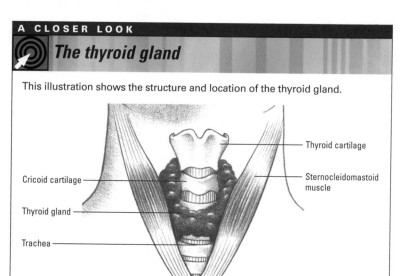

Cricoid cartilage

Thyroid gland

Trachea

Thyroid cartilage

Sternocleidomastoid muscle

drooping mouth could point to a neurologic impairment.

Next, listen to your patient's voice, noting the tone and listening for hoarseness or a nasal quality. Observe for dentures or missing teeth. Smell his breath to detect unusual odors.

Skin condition

Look at the skin surrounding his nose and mouth, noting the color of the lips and the area immediately surrounding the mouth. Discoloration or a break in skin integrity could signal a problem. Note swelling, bleeding, or drainage.

CHECKING VITAL SIGNS

Check the patient's vital signs, especially his temperature. A fever indicates infection, a common problem with complaints of the nose and throat. If you notice any sign of injury or if your patient has a nose-

bleed, pay close attention to pulse rate and blood pressure.

FOCUSING ON THE CHIEF SIGN OR SYMPTOM

After you've made general observations and checked the patient's vital signs, you'll want to focus on the patient's chief nose or throat sign or symptom for the history and physical assessment.

Further assessment

Other body systems, such as the neurologic system, may need to be assessed to completely evaluate some of these signs and symptoms. After obtaining a history and performing the physical assessment, you'll begin to form a diagnostic impression. (See *Nose and throat: Interpreting your findings.*)

DIAGNOSTIC IMPRESSION

 Nose and throat: Interpreting your findings

After you assess the patient, a group of findings may lead you to suspect a particular disorder. The chart below shows common groups of findings for the signs and symptoms of the nose and throat, along with their probable causes.

Sign or symptom and findings	Probable cause
Dysphagia	
• Signs of respiratory distress, such as crowing and stridor • Phase 2 dysphagia with gagging and dysphonia	Airway obstruction
• Phase 2 and 3 dysphagia • Rapid weight loss • Steady chest pain • Cough with hemoptysis • Hoarseness • Sore throat • Hiccups	Esophageal cancer
• Painless, progressive dysphagia • Lead line on the gums • Metallic taste • Papilledema • Ocular palsy • Footdrop or wristdrop • Mental impairment or seizures	Lead poisoning
Epistaxis	
• Ecchymoses • Petechiae • Bleeding from the gums, mouth, and I.V. puncture sites • Menorrhagia • Signs of GI bleeding, such as melena and hematemesis	Coagulation disorders
• Unilateral or bilateral epistaxis • Nasal swelling • Periorbital ecchymoses and edema • Pain • Nasal deformity • Crepitation of the nasal bones	Nasal fracture

(continued)

Nose and throat: Interpreting your findings (continued)

Sign or symptom and findings	Probable cause
Epistaxis (continued)	
• Oozing epistaxis • Dry cough • Abrupt onset of chills and high fever • "Rose-spot" rash • Vomiting • Profound fatigue • Anorexia	Typhoid fever
Nasal obstruction	
• Watery nasal discharge • Sneezing • Temporary loss of smell and taste • Sore throat • Malaise • Arthralgia • Mild headache	Common cold
• Anosmia • Clear, watery nasal discharge • History of allergies, chronic sinusitis, trauma, cystic fibrosis, or asthma • Translucent, pear-shaped polyps that are unilateral or bilateral	Nasal polyps
• Thick, purulent drainage • Severe pain over the sinuses • Fever • Inflamed nasal mucosa with purulent mucus	Sinusitis
Throat pain	
• Throat pain that occurs seasonally or year-round • Nasal congestion with a thin nasal discharge and postnasal drip • Paroxysmal sneezing • Decreased sense of smell • Frontal or temporal headache • Pale and glistening nasal mucosa with edematous nasal turbinates • Watery eyes	Allergic rhinitis

Nose and throat: Interpreting your findings (continued)

Sign or symptom and findings	Probable cause
Throat pain *(continued)*	
• Mild to severe hoarseness • Temporary loss of voice • Malaise • Low-grade fever • Dysphagia • Dry cough • Tender, enlarged cervical lymph nodes	Laryngitis
• Mild to severe sore throat • Pain may radiate to the ears • Dysphagia • Headache • Malaise • Fever with chills • Tender cervical lymphadenopathy	Tonsillitis, acute

Common signs and symptoms

A patient may seek care for any number of signs and symptoms related to the nose and throat. Some common ones are dysphagia, epistaxis, nasal obstruction, and throat pain. The following section will help you assess these signs and symptoms quickly and accurately.

DYSPHAGIA

Dysphagia is a common symptom that's usually easy to localize. It may be constant or intermittent. Among the factors that cause difficulty with swallowing are severe pain, obstruction, abnormal peristalsis, impaired gag reflex, and excessive, scanty, or thick oral secretions.

History

If the patient's dysphagia doesn't suggest airway obstruction, begin a health history. Ask the patient if swallowing is painful. If so, is the pain constant or intermittent? Have the patient point to where dysphagia feels most intense. Does eating alleviate or aggravate the symptom? Are solids or liquids more difficult to swallow? If the answer is liquids, ask if hot, cold, and lukewarm fluids affect him differently. Does the symptom disappear after he tries to swallow a few times? Is swallowing easier if he changes position? Ask if he has recently experienced vomiting, regurgitation, weight loss, anorexia, hoarseness, dyspnea, or a cough.

Physical assessment

To evaluate the patient's swallowing reflex, place your finger along his thyroid notch and instruct him to swallow. If you feel the larynx rise, the reflex is intact. Next, have him cough to assess his cough reflex. Check his gag reflex if you're sure he has a good swallow or cough reflex. Listen closely to his speech for signs of muscle weakness. Does he have aphasia or dysarthria? Is his voice nasal, hoarse, or breathy? Assess the patient's mouth carefully. Check for dry mucous membranes and thick, sticky secretions. Observe for tongue and facial weakness. Assess the patient for disorientation, which may make him neglect to swallow.

Analysis

Dysphagia is classified by the phase of swallowing it affects. Phase 1 dysphagia occurs during the transfer phase when swallowing begins, as the tongue presses against the hard palate to transfer the chewed food to the back of the throat. Phase 1 dysphagia usually results from a neuromuscular disorder. Phase 2 dysphagia occurs during the transfer phase of swallowing, when the soft palate closes against the pharyngeal wall to prevent nasal regurgitation. Phase 2 dysphagia usually indicates spasm or cancer. Phase 3 dysphagia occurs during the entrance phase of swallowing, as the food moves through the esophageal sphincter and into the stomach. Phase 3 dysphagia results from lower esophageal narrowing by diverticula, esophagitis, and other disorders.

Dysphagia is the most common (and often the only) symptom of esophageal disorders. However, it may also result from an oropharyngeal, respiratory, neurologic, or collagen disorder or from the effects of toxins and treatments. Dysphagia increases the risk of choking and aspiration and may lead to malnutrition and dehydration.

PEDIATRIC TIP

In looking for dysphagia in an infant or a small child, be sure to pay close attention to sucking and swallowing ability. Coughing, choking, or regurgitation during feeding suggests dysphagia.

Corrosive esophagitis and esophageal obstruction by a foreign body are more common causes of dysphagia in children than in adults. However, dysphagia may also result from congenital anomalies, such as annular stenosis, dysphagia lusoria, and esophageal atresia.

GERIATRIC TIP

In those older than age 50 with head or neck cancer, dysphagia is usually the first symptom that causes the patient to seek care. The incidence of such cancers increases markedly in this age-group.

EPISTAXIS

Epistaxis can be spontaneous or induced from the front or back of the nose. Most nosebleeds occur in the anterior-inferior nasal septum (Kiesselbach's plexus), but they may also occur at the point where the inferior turbinates meet the nasopharynx. Usually unilateral, they seem bilateral when blood runs from the bleeding side behind the nasal septum and out the opposite side. Epistaxis ranges from mild oozing to severe—possibly life-threatening—blood loss.

History

If your patient isn't in distress, take a history. Does he have a history of recent trauma? How often has he had nosebleeds in the past? Have the nosebleeds been long or unusually severe? Has the patient recently had surgery in the sinus area? Ask about a history of hypertension, bleeding, or liver disorders and other recent illnesses. Ask whether the patient bruises easily. Find out what drugs he uses, especially anti-inflammatories, such as aspirin, and anticoagulants such as warfarin.

Physical assessment

Begin the physical examination by inspecting the patient's skin for other signs of bleeding, such as ecchymoses and petechiae, and noting jaundice, pallor, or other abnormalities. When examining a trauma patient, look for associated injuries, such as eye trauma or facial fractures.

If your patient has severe epistaxis, quickly take his vital signs. Be alert for tachypnea, hypotension, and other signs of hypovolemic shock. Attempt to control bleeding by pinching the nares closed. Have a hypovolemic patient lie down and turn his head to the side to prevent blood from draining down the back of the throat, which could cause aspiration or vomiting of swallowed blood. If the patient isn't hypovolemic, have him sit upright and tilt his head forward. Constantly check airway patency.

Analysis

A rich supply of fragile blood vessels makes the nose particularly vulnerable to bleeding. Air moving through the nose can dry and irritate the mucous membranes, forming crusts that bleed when they're removed; dry mucous membranes are also more susceptible to infection, which can produce epistaxis as well. Trauma is another common cause of epistaxis. Additional causes include septal deviations; hematologic, coagulation, renal, and GI disorders; and certain drugs and treatments.

PEDIATRIC TIP

Children are more likely to experience anterior nosebleeds, usually the result of nose picking or allergic rhinitis. Biliary atresia, cystic fibrosis, hereditary afibrinogenemia, and nasal trauma due to a foreign body can also cause epistaxis. Rubeola may cause an oozing nosebleed along with the characteristic maculopapular rash. Two rare childhood diseases—pertussis and diphtheria—can also cause oozing epistaxis.

Suspect a bleeding disorder if you see excess umbilical cord bleeding at birth or profuse bleeding during circumcision. Epistaxis usually begins at puberty in patients with hereditary hemorrhagic telangiectasia.

GERIATRIC TIP

Elderly patients are more likely to have posterior nosebleeds.

NASAL OBSTRUCTION

Rarely a serious problem, obstruction of the nasal mucous membranes may be either self-limiting or chronic.

History

Begin the history by asking the patient about the duration and frequency of the obstruction. Did it begin suddenly or gradually? Is it intermittent or persistent? Unilateral or bilateral? Inquire about the presence and character of drainage. Is it watery, purulent, or bloody? Does the patient have nasal or sinus pain or headaches? Ask about recent travel, the use of drugs or alcohol, and previous trauma or surgery.

Physical assessment

Examine the patient's nose; assess airflow and the condition of the turbinates and nasal septum. Evaluate the orbits for evidence of dystopia, decreased vision, excess tearing, or abnormal appearance of the eye. Palpate over the frontal and maxillary sinuses for tenderness. Examine the ears for signs of middle ear effusions. Inspect the oral cavity, pharynx, nasopharynx, and larynx to detect inflammation, ulceration, excessive mucosal dryness, and neurologic deficits. Lastly, palpate the neck for adenopathy.

Analysis

Nasal obstruction may result from an inflammatory, neoplastic, endocrine, or metabolic disorder; a structural abnormality; or a traumatic injury. It may cause discomfort, alter a person's sense of taste and smell, and cause voice changes. Although a frequent and typically benign symptom, nasal obstruction may herald certain life-threatening disorders, such as a basilar skull fracture or a malignant tumor.

PEDIATRIC TIP

Acute nasal obstruction in children usually results from the common cold. In infants and children, especially between ages 3 and 6, chronic nasal obstruction typically results from large adenoids. In neonates, choanal atresia is the most common congenital cause of nasal obstruction and can be unilateral or bilateral. Cystic fibrosis may cause nasal polyps in children, resulting in nasal obstruction. However, if the child has unilateral nasal obstruction and rhinorrhea, you should assume a foreign body in the nose until proven otherwise.

THROAT PAIN

Throat pain—commonly known as a sore throat—refers to discomfort in any part of the pharynx: the nasopharynx, the oropharynx, or the hypopharynx. This common symptom ranges from a sensation of scratchiness to severe pain. It's typically accompanied by ear pain because cranial nerves IX and X innervate the pharynx as well as the middle and external ear.

History

Ask the patient when he first noticed the pain, and have him describe it. Has he had throat pain before? Is it accompanied by fever, ear pain, or dysphagia? Review the patient's medical history for throat problems, allergies, and systemic disorders.

Physical assessment

Carefully examine the pharynx, noting redness, exudate, or swelling. Examine the oropharynx, using a warmed metal spatula or tongue blade, and the nasopharynx, using a warmed laryngeal mirror or a fiber-optic nasopharyngoscope. Laryngoscopic examination of the hypopharynx may be required. (If necessary, spray the soft palate and pharyngeal wall with a local anesthetic to prevent gagging.) Observe the tonsils for redness, swelling, or exudate. In addition, obtain an exudate specimen for culture. Then examine the nose, using a nasal speculum. Also, check the patient's ears, especially if he reports ear pain. Finally, palpate the neck and oropharynx for nodules or lymph node enlargement.

Analysis

Throat pain may result from infection, trauma, allergy, cancer, and certain systemic disorders. It may also follow surgery and endotracheal intubation. Nonpathologic causes include dry mucous membranes associated with mouth breathing and laryngeal irritation associated with alcohol consumption, inhaling smoke or chemicals like ammonia, and vocal strain.

PEDIATRIC TIP

Sore throat is a common complaint in children and may result from many of the same disorders that affect adults. Other pediatric causes of sore throat include acute epiglottitis, herpangina, scarlet fever, acute follicular tonsillitis, and retropharyngeal abscess.

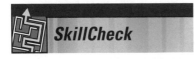

SkillCheck

1. Which symptom commonly accompanies throat pain?
   a. Eye pain
   b. Ear pain
   c. Headache
   d. Nasal congestion

Answer: b. Ear pain, because cranial nerves IX and X innervate the pharynx as well as the middle and external ear, throat pain and ear pain commonly occur together.

2. If your patient presents with severe epistaxis, what's important for you to check quickly?
   a. His history
   b. His height
   c. His weight
   d. His vital signs

Answer: d. After pinching the nose to stop the bleeding, you should check your patient's vital signs for tachypnea and hypotension—signs of hypovolemic shock.

3. What's the most common symptom of an esophageal disorder?
   a. Epistaxis
   b. Nasal obstruction
   c. Dysphagia
   d. Throat pain

Answer: c. Dysphagia is the most common, and sometimes the only, symptom of an esophageal disorder, such as esophageal cancer or esophageal diverticulum.

4. If your patient complains of pain as he begins to swallow food, which phase of dysphagia would you classify this as?
   a. Phase 1
   b. Phase 2
   c. Phase 3
   d. Phase 4

Answer: a. Pain when food is being passed to the back of the throat, at the transfer phase of swallowing, should be classified as Phase 1 dysphagia.

5. Which cause of nasal obstruction is life-threatening?
   a. Basilar skull fracture
   b. Common cold
   c. Nasal polyps
   d. Sinusitis

Answer: a. A basilar skull fracture is life-threatening and can lead to cerebrospinal rhinorrhea with nasal obstruction.

Domestic abuse assessment

Domestic violence is abuse by a caregiver, a parent, a spouse, or an intimate partner. There are many forms of abuse including physical, sexual, verbal, and emotional abuse, as well as control of access to money and control of activities.

Screening of all patients for domestic abuse should be a routine part of your assessment whether signs, symptoms, or behaviors suggest the presence of abuse or not. Simply asking questions is an intervention. Even if abuse isn't disclosed, it reassures the patient that you're concerned and if needed there's a safe place to go in the future.

Some states require reporting current victimization to law enforcement or social services. Follow the laws in your state and tell the patient about any limits of confidentiality before conducting your assessment. Identified abuse of children, elders, and disabled persons by law must be reported to state protection agencies. However, all domestic violence requires appropriate assessment and intervention by the practitioner.

It's important that policies, protocol, and practice regarding the use of information you obtain in your assessment are in place to maintain patient confidentiality.

Screening tips

- Screen patients when you're alone with them (except children under 3). Defer the assessment if the practitioner can't secure a private space to conduct the screening.
- Ask family and friends to wait in the waiting area during history taking and screening.
- Conduct the screening face to face.
- Include written or computer-based health questionnaires when appropriate.
- Use nonjudgmental language that's culturally appropriate.
- Maintain confidentiality; inform the patient of any reporting requirements before starting the assessment.
- If an interpreter is necessary, ensure that they've been trained to ask about abuse and that they don't know the patient or the patient's partner, caregiver, friends, or family. Defer the assessment if an appropriate interpreter isn't available.
- Actively listen, show concern, and provide validation.
- Reassure the patient that the disclosure won't be reported back to the abuser.
- If the screening environment is unsafe for either the patient or the health care provider, defer the screening until a safe environment is secured.

TYPICAL QUESTIONS TO ASK

- Do you ever feel unsafe or threatened by anyone?
- Have you ever been afraid of anyone?
- Has anyone ever hurt you or someone you care about?
- Is anyone trying to control you—who you see and talk to, where you go, what you wear, how you spend money?
- How does your partner act when angry?
- This injury doesn't look like it came from a fall; are you sure that's how this happened?
- Can you talk to me about what's happening at home?

BARRIERS TO DISCLOSING DOMESTIC VIOLENCE

Several factors may prevent a patient from disclosing abuse including:

- fear that the health care provider will judge them
- fear of threats by the abuser that harm will come if abuse is disclosed
- lack of confidence in the system
- fear that no one will believe the abuse is happening
- fear of blame for staying in the abusive situation or for not reporting sooner
- inability to be aware abuse is occurring or the patient doesn't know how to talk about abuse
- minimization of the seriousness of "domestic abuse"
- lack of financial or social independence.

DOCUMENTATION TIPS

Medical records are often the best and only documentation of abuse that can be used in court. Be detailed, objective, and legible when you document. If your assessment conflicts with the patient's report, note the difference. Include:

- date and time of the suspected abuse
- the patient's account, specific details, injuries sustained, and weapons used, if any
- history of previous abuse
- a description of physical findings and body mapping of injuries when applicable
- the practitioner's assessment, recommendations, information provided, and safety planning
- resources and referrals provided
- documentation of mandatory reporting of child, disabled, or elder abuse.

Selected references

Assessment Made Incredibly Easy, 3rd ed. Philadelphia: Lippincott Williams & Wilkins, 2005.

Assessment: A 2-in-1 Reference for Nurses. Philadelphia: Lippincott Williams & Wilkins, 2005.

Bickley, L.S., and Szilagyi, P.G. *Bates' Guide to Physical Examination and History Taking,* 9th ed. Philadelphia: Lippincott Williams & Wilkins, 2007.

Hogstel, M.O., and Curry, L.C. *Practical Guide to Health Assessment: Through the Life Span,* 4th ed. Philadelphia: F.A. Davis Co., 2005.

Jarvis, C. *Physical Examination and Health Assessment,* 4th ed. Philadelphia: W.B. Saunders Co., 2004.

Linton, A.D. *Introduction to Medical-Surgical Nursing,* 3rd ed. Philadelphia: W.B. Saunders Co., 2003.

Nutrition Made Incredibly Easy, 2nd ed. Philadelphia: Lippincott Williams & Wilkins, 2007.

Potter, P.A., and Perry, A.G. *Fundamentals of Nursing,* 6th ed. St. Louis: Mosby–Year Book, Inc., 2005.

Professional Guide to Signs & Symptoms, 5th ed. Philadelphia: Lippincott Williams & Wilkins, 2006.

Smeltzer, S.C., and Bare, B.G. *Brunner and Suddarth's Textbook of Medical-Surgical Nursing,* 10th ed. Philadelphia: Lippincott Williams & Wilkins, 2004.

Weber, J.R. *Nurses' Handbook of Health Assessment,* 5th ed. Philadelphia: Lippincott Williams & Wilkins, 2005.

Index

i refers to an illustration; t refers to a table.

i refers to an illustration; t refers to a table.